"Outstanding manual that offers a comprehensive approach to change that covers the major area. of anxiety. Uniquely emphasizes the links between anxiety and common co-occurring conditions, such as procrastination and indecision. The book shows how to combat anxiety cognitions, build emotional tolerance, use imagery for relaxation, engage in problem-solving behaviors, and apply tested techniques for solving more than one emotional problem simultaneously. It features self-contracts at the end of each chapter to reinforce change."

—**Janet Wolfe, PhD**, former executive director of the Albert Ellis Institute and staff psychologist for thirty-five years, as well as author or coauthor of multiple books, including *What to Do When He Has a Headache*

"This book is brilliant! Scientifically sound, user-friendly, compassionate, and deeply understanding of the anxiety disorders—I will insist that many of my patients read it. In fact, regular use of Knaus's workbook may actually shorten the length of time required for some anxiety sufferers to remain in therapy."

—**Barry Lubetkin, PhD, ABPP**, director and founder of the Institute for Behavior Therapy, New York City

"Knaus has an amazing capacity to simplify and clarify complex scientific ideas and to incorporate them into an accessible, pragmatic text. This workbook can greatly benefit lay people afflicted with excessive anxiety and commonly associated disturbances. He has added a section on meditative practices, which greatly enhances the appeal and utility of this workbook. I recommend it heartily."

—**Joseph Gerstein, MD, FACP**, founding president of the SMART Recovery Self-Help Network

"As we strive to navigate the waves of change, push ourselves to constantly do better, and struggle to accomplish a sense of balance, we can fall prey to the ravages of fear, anxiety, and depression. Knaus impresses once again by providing a highly practical, research-based methodology to tackle these psychological demons. Readers will come away with useful tools and strategies that will allow them to take charge of their lives, restore their well-being, and advance their health and productivity. Practitioners will also find this workbook a valuable and indispensable resource."

—**Sam Klarreich, PhD, C Psych**, president of The Berkeley Center for Effectiveness and The Center for Rational Emotive Therapy, and coauthor of *Fearless Job Hunting*

"One of the foundational tenets of the cognitive behavioral therapies is that personal change does not take place in the therapist's office. Rather, a patient can only make desired change by practicing—yes, practicing—the insights and strategies the therapist provides in the context of his or her daily life. Bill Knaus's *The Cognitive Behavioral Workbook for Anxiety* is a rare gem in this regard; it is both a reference for the therapist to guide the patient through the anxiety-defeating change process and also a suitable resource for the layperson to independently obliterate anxiety on his or her own. I will treasure it for my own personal use, keep copies on hand for my anxious patients as an adjunct for their therapy, and make participants aware of it at my self-help workshops.

> —**Russ Greiger, PhD**, clinical psychologist in private practice in Charlottesville, VA, and coauthor of *Fearless Job Hunting*

"Working through each page of *The Cognitive Behavioral Workbook for Anxiety* will empower any reader who is truly ready to get down to the heart of the matter! In this excellent and comprehensive collection of our current understandings and research-driven techniques, Knaus reveals a full and user-friendly plan for the great defeat of anxiety-feeding beliefs and habits!"

> —**Pam Garcy, PhD**, psychologist in Dallas, TX, and author of *The REBT Super Activity Guide*

"Knaus's step-by-step approach to conquer anxiety is written in a manner that gives the reader a handle on the source of his or her anxiety and spells out a plethora of sensible, evidence-based solutions. I heartily recommend *The Cognitive Behavioral Workbook for Anxiety* to anyone struggling with worry, anxiety, procrastination, and depression. If getting a better handle on emotions, giving up perfectionism, and defeating social anxiety are your goals, Knaus's book will seem as though he wrote it with you in mind."

> —**Joel Block, PhD**, assistant clinical professor, Hofstra, North-Shore/LIJ School of Medicine

"A fantastic tool for all those who struggle with anxiety and want to learn how to reduce it once and for all. Knaus has compiled a very practical, clear, and effective workbook, complemented by catchy, easy-to-remember tips and a very comprehensive coverage of anti-anxiety strategies and techniques following in the footsteps of Dr. Albert Ellis's theory of rational emotive behavior therapy. I will recommend this workbook to all my anxiety patients."

> —**Roberta Galluccio Richardson, PhD**, clinical psychologist, Sloane Medical Practice, London

"In this recent revision, Knaus has provided the reader with an up-to-date and comprehensive description of anxiety and the role it can play in our now all-too-complicated and demanding lives. More importantly, he gives the reader those essential and valuable tools he or she needs to better cope with and reduce modern day stress and anxiety. I strongly recommend this book to the lay reader and professional alike. This book is truly a gem!"

—**Allen Elkin, PhD**, in private practice in New York, NY, and author of *Stress Management for Dummies*

"Knaus has given us an extensive new edition of his highly successful *The Cognitive Behavioral Workbook for Anxiety*. From direct observation, we know that the completion of this project has been a labor of love. Knaus has a strong scientist-clinician's grasp of the topics he covers in this revised edition, and it shows! Throughout the book, he shares his clinical insights and thorough understanding of the anxiety research. This book effectively summarizes many approaches to coping with anxiety and offers help to those who needlessly suffer its effects. It is a goldmine of proven ways and innovative methods to cope with the many faces of anxiety. The self-helper who chooses to reduce or end needless anxieties and fears, regardless of the form that they take, will find an organized approach for developing the skills needed to manage anxiety or make it go away."

—**Leon Pomeroy, PhD**, author of *The New Science of Axiological Psychology* and **Wendy Pomeroy, MD**, US Department of Justice, retired

"Knaus's *The Cognitive Behavioral Workbook for Anxiety* is a well-constructed, thoughtful exploration of both the causes of and approaches to overcoming or minimizing anxiety and its effects. His book clearly illustrates the principles and particular steps involved in overcoming anxiety. In addition, each chapter provides clearly delineated, practical steps to address the principle causes of anxiety as the subject of each chapter. I have found the approach to addressing 'double trouble' particularly useful with clients and friends alike. Oftentimes, simply pointing out how 'awfulizing' about having anxiety brings almost immediate relief and allows the person to focus on the circumstances and causes of their anxiety. It is clear to me that fully deploying the exercises found in his workbook will bring benefit to almost anyone struggling with the ill-effects of anxiety."

—**James W. Thompson, PhD, MBA**, business psychologist

"Knaus's excellent book on overcoming anxiety just got even more versatile with this new improved edition. A virtual one-stop supermarket of information, techniques, case illustrations, top tips, and exercises for overcoming debilitating anxiety and worry, this fully revised and updated resource serves multiple purposes. From the unhappy traveler of life looking to feel and do better, to the therapist in search of an innovative and creative cognitive behavioral approach, this book serves them all—and incredibly well. Knaus has truly outdone himself on this one!"

—**Elliot D. Cohen, PhD**, author of *What would Aristotle Do? Self-Control through the Power of Reason*

"Anxiety is so common that almost everyone experiences it from time to time. It can interfere with fully living the only life you have to live. Knaus, a renowned cognitive behavioral therapist and author, has summarized the cutting-edge knowledge and provided practical steps for you to follow to deal with anxiety. By following this precious wisdom, you can gain relief from the suffering caused by anxiety."

—**Sanjay Singh, MD, DNB, PhD**, REBT and REE representative in India, professor, Department of Dermatology, Institute of Medical Sciences, Banaras Hindu University, Varanasi, India.

"If you want to reduce and control your anxieties, worries, fears, etc., Socrates's advice still holds: 'Know yourself!' But how do you do it? Even small steps can help, and this workbook by veteran psychotherapist Knaus will guide you along the way with a variety of practical tools you can immediately apply for observing and managing your thinking-feeling-acting. Alfred Korzybski, an early pioneer in what is now called cognitive behavioral therapy, said fears and defensiveness *are no defense*. You can learn how to manage yours."

—**Bruce I. Kodish**, author of *Korzybski: A Biography* and *Drive Yourself Sane: Using the Uncommon Sense of General Semantics*, coauthored with Susan Presby Kodish

"Freud distinguished between fearing what is harmful and threatening to our survival (realistic anxiety) and all other fears (neurotic anxiety). Knaus offers systematic ways to reduce self-handicapping unrealistic anxieties with a series of exercises and written progress reports. Building on decades of work in cognitive behavioral therapy, he presents highly practical and creative ideas for educating oneself against anxiety and toward a calmer, more comfortable, and productive life. His is a valuable, no-nonsense approach to self-help."

—**Richard L. Wessler, PhD**, emeritus professor of psychology and codeveloper of cognitive appraisal therapy

"Knaus has done it again with an important update to his best-selling book *The Cognitive Behavioral Workbook for Anxiety*. Not only is this a self-help manual, but it could also be used as a college textbook in a counseling psychology course. It is astonishingly well written, and the coverage is detailed and thorough. As a self-help manual it offers a clear, step-by-step solution to the dilemma of depression and anxiety. It gets the reader moving and changing, because it demands that the reader be involved enough to take active steps. This is not for the passively disengaged, but for those who are willing to participate in their own recovery process (which is essential to the overall healing). As a textbook it is a foundational source for a true understanding of cognitive behavioral therapy, which has been proven to be today's most effective therapeutic technique. And in this case you will be reading words from the master, as Knaus himself has contributed greatly to the creation of this important therapeutic breakthrough."

—**Richard Sprinthall, PhD**, emeritus professor at American International College

"This revision of Knaus's *Cognitive Behavioral Work Book for Anxiety* is no less than a milestone in the CBT self-help movement. It is both a compassionate and scholarly reach-out to all those suffering from anxieties that thwart their well-being and development. I am sure, given my personal acquaintance with the founding fathers of CBT, such as Albert Ellis, that they also would applaud the publication of this helpful volume."

—**René F.W. Diekstra, PhD**, emeritus professor of psychology at the University College in Roosevelt Middelburg, the Netherlands, and professor of youth and development at the University of Applied Sciences at The Hague, the Netherlands

The Cognitive Behavioral Workbook *for* Anxiety

SECOND EDITION

A STEP-BY-STEP PROGRAM

WILLIAM J. KNAUS, EdD

New Harbinger Publications, Inc.

Publisher's Note

Distributed in Canada by Raincoast Books

Copyright © 2014 by William J. Knaus
               New Harbinger Publications, Inc.
               5674 Shattuck Avenue
               Oakland, CA 94609
               www.newharbinger.com

Cover design by Amy Shoup
Acquired by Jess O'Brien
Edited by Brady Kahn

Library of Congress Cataloging-in-Publication Data

Knaus, William J.
  The cognitive behavioral workbook for anxiety : a step-by-step program / William J. Knaus, EdD ; foreword by Jon Carlson, PsyD, EdD, ABPP. -- Second edition.
    pages cm
  Includes bibliographical references and index.
  ISBN 978-1-62625-015-4 (paperback) -- ISBN 978-1-62625-016-1 (pdf e-book) -- ISBN 978-1-62625-017-8 (epub) 1. Anxiety--Treatment. 2. Rational emotive behavior therapy. 3. Cognitive therapy. I. Title.
  RC531.K63 2014
  616.85'2206--dc23
                2014017718

Printed in the United States of America

18   17   16

10   9   8   7   6   5   4

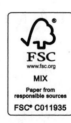
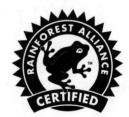

Contents

Acknowledgments

I'd like to acknowledge the following people for their marvelous contributions and helpful tips to the readers of this book:

Dr. Bob Alberti, Dr. Irwin Altrows, Dr. Judith Beck, Dr. Joel Block, Dr. Elliot Cohen, Dr. Daniel David, Dr. Pam Garcy, Ed Garcia, Dr. William Golden, Michael Gregory, Dr. Russ Grieger, Dr. Steven Hayes, Dale Jarvis, Dr. Howie Kassinove, Dr. Sam Klarreich, Dr. Cliff Lazarus, Dr. John Minor, Dr. George Morelli, Dr. Ron Murphy, Dr. John Norcross, Dr. Rick Paar, Dr. Vince Parr, Will Ross, Dr. Jeff Rudolph, Justin Rudolph, Dr. Jack Shannon, Dr. Susan Krauss Whitbourne, and especially my wife, Dr. Nancy Knaus who reviewed this book as it was in process and who contributed a tip on preventing anxiety.

Foreword

My grandparents, who emigrated directly from Sweden, used to tell me, "Worry gives a small thing a big shadow." Many habits of the mind are transferred to us through this kind of transgenerational learning. Some learnings help us to cope with life, while others—including fears, anxieties, and phobias—tend to be destructive.

Alfred Adler explained that anxiety has a purpose: it is a safeguarding mechanism that causes us to frighten ourselves out of doing things. We could simply decide not to do these things, but then we might have to face our complexes and admit to having them. With anxiety as a mechanism, we claim we are too afraid to try (Carlson, Watts, and Maniacci 2006). These patterns frequently arise without our direct awareness or conscious intent.

Anxiety affects one-third of the population at one time or another. A web search turns up nearly 60 million entries for anxiety alone. The various listings describe the many strategies purported to provide relief. These range from drugs to biblical passages to diets to folk cures.

This best-selling book stands out in that it offers strategies that have been researched and proven effective. They do not promise a quick fix but rather teach us how to take responsibility for our own lives. Too many people blame others for their personal challenges. As Bill Knaus states, "Blame, like the air, is everywhere." This book provides three basic prescriptions to help conquer the problem of anxiety:

1. Educate your reason to oppose parasitic thinking and reacting. (Change your thoughts.)

2. Learn to build emotional tolerance. (Strengthen your emotions.)

3. Behaviorally engage the fear and desensitize yourself to it. (Take action.)

The fact that these interventions integrate thinking, feeling, and acting modalities allows readers to utilize their unique strengths and preferences.

The quickest way to clear anxiety out of your body is to take a few deep belly breaths. Chest breathing seems to be wired into anxiety production, while belly breathing is connected to anxiety reduction. If you are anxious, you can wait until you are not anxious, and your breathing will slow down. But if you are in a hurry to clear out the anxiety, you can consciously slow down your breathing and watch the anxiety go away.

By concentrating on our breathing, we create a sense of serenity. We can learn to accept the fact of fear, learn to feel fear fully, and learn to thrive by acting in a manner that prevents fear from interfering with life choices. As David Richo (2008, 21–22) states, "We all feel afraid sometimes. This is an appropriate feeling and can be a signal of real danger and threat. At the same time, we sometimes feel afraid without reason. Our guesses and fantasies about what might happen keep us afraid of events and experiences that may never befall us. It is useless to attempt to eliminate fear altogether, whether it be ritualistic or imagined."

This revised book adds to the original impressive collection of techniques that can be used to provide the courage necessary to face anxieties and fears. Dr. Knaus also offers thirty-two "quick tips" contributed by today's leading anxiety experts. All of the strategies have their roots in the work of the great psychologists Alfred Adler, Aaron Beck, Albert Ellis, and Arnold Lazarus and have withstood the test of time. They can change transgenerational learning patterns by helping readers develop courage and self-control.

The profession of psychology has advanced in the short time since the original edition of this book appeared. The completely revised book remains a most valuable resource for therapists and their clients who wish to learn cutting-edge methods of anxiety treatment. This new edition is more than a self-help book for anxiety. Readers will learn to not only eliminate anxieties and fears but also prevent their return. Additionally, the book provides a program for developing the self-efficacy, serenity, confidence, and control needed for living a satisfying life overall.

As I read through this exceptional resource book, I am reminded of the power of the mind. Bill Knaus has clearly presented many effective strategies that will allow readers to solve their own problems. This type of solution will lead to the greater psychological hardiness and self-efficacy of the population. It is now possible to go beyond our many self-imposed prisons. Eleanor Roosevelt said it best: "You must do the things you think you cannot do."

—Jon Carlson, PsyD, EdD, ABPP
Distinguished Professor
Division of Psychology and Counseling
Governors State University

Introduction

Do you sometimes feel overwhelmed by your anxieties and fears? Does one misery follow another? Do you hold to lofty ideals and feel anxious about falling short? Do you actively avoid whatever you fear even when you know the fear is silly?

Few go through life without having their share of irrational anxieties and fears; some have more than their fair share. Some of these anxieties are like reoccurring storms. But unlike weather patterns that you can't change, you can do many things to change the intensity, duration, and course of your anxieties and fears.

You are not crazy for having anxieties. You may have a sensitive fear signaling system and startle easily. You may feel anxious or fearful about having sensations such as an increased heart rate, sweating, and tension headaches. The issue isn't whether you have fears or anxieties; the issue is, what can you do to liberate yourself from needless fears and anxieties? Cognitive behavioral therapy (CBT) methods are effective for curbing both.

Here's the idea. Your cognitions (thoughts, mental images, memories), emotions, and behaviors blend together. Changes in one of these areas affect the others. Thus, if you no longer see a situation as threatening, your anxiety drops. You may approach what you formerly feared. That's the anxiety solution. The cognitive behavioral changes that you make are relatively durable (Gloster et al. 2013).

Here is a question you should be asking yourself: Where's the evidence that CBT is effective against anxiety?

CBT RESEARCH

Over the past forty years, CBT has amassed strong evidence to show effectiveness for reducing and ending disturbing conditions, such as anxiety and depression (Öst 2008).

- Meta-analyses affirm CBT's general effectiveness (Butler et al. 2006) and specifically for combatting anxiety (Olatunji, Cisler, and Deacon 2010).

- A survey of 269 CBT meta-analyses shows that the system is effective for people suffering from a broad range of problems, such as substance abuse, depression, and anxiety. The results point to CBT as a consistently strong method for reducing anxiety (Hofmann et al. 2012).

- Specific studies demonstrate that you can use CBT for decreasing anxious ruminations (Reinecke et al. 2013), for reducing panic (Rayburn and Otto 2003), for overcoming social anxieties (Furukawa et al. 2013), and for toning down those parts of your brain's artificial anxiety and fear generating network (Kircher et al. 2013).

- CBT is a brain training method. Healthy brain function and brain structural changes are observed after CBT (Collerton 2013).

- The CBT system is a strong alternative to the anxiolytic and hypnotic drugs used to medically treat anxiety. This class of drugs is addictive and associated with increased mortality (Weich et al. 2014).

- CBT is viewed as the gold standard for treating anxiety (Otte 2011).

Throughout this book you'll find references to articles and research studies. They are illustrative, not exhaustive, which means you could have long lists of studies for most referenced topics. They help answer the question, "Where's the evidence?"

Healing Through Reading

Can a CBT bibliotherapy approach (healing through reading) work? A self-help book that relies on evidence-based CBT methods can help you decrease your anxieties (Hirai and Clum 2006). Highly rated psychology self-help books are written by doctoral level mental health professionals and deal with specific problems (Redding et al. 2008). Books that show how to cope with conditions that commonly occur with anxiety, such as self-image problems and fear of the feeling of fear, may be the wave of the future (Craske 2012).

The future is now. What you learn through your self-help efforts can produce favorable results. But know your limitations. You don't have to travel this road alone. When appropriate, enlist the help of a CBT therapist or compassionate and helpful friend.

Plan to move at a pace that is reasonable for you. Don't expect overnight success. Rapid changes do occur, but this is more the exception than the rule.

"Skill to do comes of doing; knowledge comes by eyes always open and working hands; and there is no knowledge that is not power"(Emerson 1870, 287). In part, the effectiveness of a psychological self-help approach lies in deepening your self-knowledge by taking action to solve your problems.

OVERCOMING MULTIPLE PROBLEMS SIMULTANEOUSLY

Most people who suffer from recurring anxieties and fears find themselves challenged by other distressful conditions (Gadermann et al. 2012). Some have connecting links. Look closely at your anxiety patterns. Do you think you are powerless to cope? Such *powerlessness thinking* is involved in anxiety, depression, and post-traumatic shock. By acting to overcome powerlessness thinking, you can ease multiple conditions that are connected to this belief that you are powerless to cope.

Likewise, you can use relaxation to address anxiety. With a calmer body, you also may find yourself worrying less. By reducing your tendency to worry, you will feel less anxious too. In other words, you often can address multiple emotional problems simultaneously by taking what is technically called a *transdiagnostic approach*, when an intervention helps to address more than just one condition.

The issue, of course, is to determine which interventions can bring about changes in multiple areas. The research on transdiagnostic approaches, while still in its infancy, is promising.

Cognitive behavioral therapy is a transdiagnostic approach that you can confidently use for anxiety. For example, CBT techniques for addressing one form of anxiety can simultaneously quiet other forms of anxiety (McEvoy et al. 2013). Certain techniques for alleviating anxiety can quell a co-occurring depression (Beck and Dozois 2011). You commonly find a combination of perfectionism, anxiety, and eating disorders (Fairburn et al. 2009), and addressing perfectionism can have a transdiagnostic effect on the other issues. Threat sensitivity can spread over many forms of anxiety (Bar-Haim et al. 2007), and teaching yourself to be less stress sensitive can decrease feelings of anxiety.

Achieving multiple benefits from a few productive interventions is appealing. But what happens if you overcome one problem anxiety, but others remain? For example, if you no longer fear small animals, but you retain a public-speaking anxiety?

Psychologist Albert Ellis's ABCDE method for changing negative thinking and taking positive action is an original transdiagnostic method that applies to practically every self-defeating cognitive, emotive, and behavioral condition (see chapter 11). If you successfully use it to overcome one anxiety, you can apply what you learned to another. As you improve in the use of this method, you may use it less often, because you will have fewer anxiety problems to address.

Psychological Homework Assignments

Psychological homework assignments are a central part of Ellis's (2000) rational emotive behavior therapy (REBT) foundation system for CBT. Psychological homework is a standard CBT practice—a transdiagnostic technique that may be especially useful when it comes to combatting your anxieties and fears. For example, if you suffer from panic and agoraphobia, doing homework assignments to face what you fear frequently reduces both conditions (Cammin-Nowak et al. 2013). Following through on psychological homework assignments correlates with self-improvement (Lebeau et al. 2013).

If you set weekly goals and give yourself assignments for meeting these goals, and you make a good-faith effort to follow through, the odds are that you'll get better results and improve more quickly than if you simply stay on the sidelines wringing your hands.

WHERE THIS BOOK WILL TAKE YOU

The Cognitive Behavioral Workbook for Anxiety (second edition) delivers step-by-step guidance for addressing parasitic anxieties and fears. You'll find multiple ideas along with multiple exercises for addressing them. More specifically, you'll find the following:

- A well-referenced book that draws from both classical and recent thinking on how to overcome anxieties and fears. The major sources for this book are cited at the end, where there is also a list of suggested reading material.

- Interventions that I've used with my clients that they found to be effective. Over the past forty-five years, I've developed numerous interventions and have selected others from the literature. By having multiple choices available, you can configure a program that works best for you.

- Learn to apply CBT self-improvement methods in different contexts (generalization) to debunk false anxiety assumptions, build tolerance for tension, and gain mastery over yourself. You'll find basic technique that apply to different problems and multiple techniques that apply to a specific anxiety. If you miss a key idea in one chapter, you are likely to see a related use later.

- Special tips from anxiety experts. I invited a group of top anxiety experts to contribute their favorite tips. Their tips throughout the book give you different perspectives on what you might do to overcome your anxieties and fears.

- Written exercises for self-improvement. Journaling and writing can be used for developing perspective, regulating emotions, and improving your psychological outlook (Stockdale 2011). Writing out problems is a therapeutic intervention that can help reduce needless tension (Van Emmerik, Kamphuis, and Emmelkamp 2008). Writing in the first person is associated with higher levels of self-improvement (Seih, Chung, and Pennebaker 2011).

I divided this workbook into four parts. Part I introduces the world of anxieties and fears. It will show you how to separate real from imagined fears and how to use basic cognitive, emotive, and behavioral ways to overcome these conditions. It will show you how to break a vicious cycle of anxiety using objective self-observation skills, how to stop escalating your anxieties, how to make progress using a self-management approach, and how to get past procrastination barriers that can interfere with positive change.

Part II shows how to use nature scenes to achieve serenity, how to relax your body, how to regulate emotions that are triggered by cognitions, how to use a classic ABCDE model to combat anxiety, and how to use key behavioral methods for overcoming fear.

Part III explores how to break patterns of worry, manage anxiety over uncertainty, calm unpleasant physical sensations, overcome panic, combat phobias, and mount a multimodal attack against anxiety and fear.

Part IV looks at how to defuse anxiety-evoking expectations, defeat harmful inhibitions, overcome anxieties you may have about yourself, earn freedom from painful social anxieties, and overcome mixed anxiety and depression. The final chapter will help you learn how to preserve the gains you've made.

How fast can you proceed with your anxiety solution program? Your pace will depend in part on where you are on this healing path. You may have already started to address your anxieties. It also will depend on your network of complications (we all have them); these networks sprout from core issues, such as a vulnerability to anxiety that is reflected in negative thinking and worry. Your pace will also depend on whether you tend to procrastinate. For example, you may wait for motivation to come out of the blue. If so, you'll be waiting a long time.

Luckily, even the most complex and painfully recurring anxieties and fears have simple and manageable features. Start with what you can manage. Build from there. But don't put off starting.

EXERCISE: WHAT IS YOUR MOST PRESSING ANXIETY?

The Chinese philosopher Lao Tzu sagely said, "The journey of a thousand miles starts from beneath your feet." As a first step in moving from stillness to action, write down your most pressing anxiety in the space provided here.

There is no one psychological antianxiety intervention that works for all people under all conditions. As you go through this program, you'll find many ways to address anxiety problems. Choose and use the best approaches for you to develop self-mastery, which can be the biggest payoff.

PART I

Basic Techniques to Defeat Anxiety and Fear

- Take a test and discover your anxiety hot spots (and where to go to get solutions).

- Learn to separate real anxieties and fears from the fictional or exaggerated kind.

- See how to manage a combined real-and-imagined threat situation.

- Start yourself on a cognitive, emotive, and behavioral path to calm your anxieties.

- Break anxiety cycles before they get out of hand.

- Substitute positive self-observant skills for catastrophic thinking.

- Discover how to build confident composure.

- Take seven steps to stop emotionally troubling yourself.

- Follow a six-phase approach for getting control over your anxieties and fears.

- Evaluate your progress with a simple three-step method.

- Use procrastination technology to follow through on overcoming your anxieties and fears.

- Free yourself from needless anxieties by resolving a tricky double-agenda dilemma.

CHAPTER 1

Welcome to the World of Anxieties and Fears

When fear causes you to escape a life-threatening danger, it is your friend. But some fears have this sordid tale to tell.

> *I am fear. I make your mind spin out of control. I wind your body tight as a drum.*
> *You try to hide from me. I will find you. Look over your shoulder. I am behind you. Look forward.*
> *My shadow crosses your path. Look into a mirror and you see me sneering back at you.*

Your exaggerated anxieties and fears drain your time and resources and offer nothing of positive value in return, which is why this book refers to them as *parasitic*. As Mark Twain once said, "I am an old man and have known a great many troubles, but most of them never happened."

When you suffer from fear and anxiety, it can be hard to imagine a different way of being. But eliminating fear and anxiety is something you can progressively do. It may help to start this journey through the eyes of some people who turned their own anxieties and fears into fading memories.

YOU ARE NOT ALONE

You are not unique when it comes to having anxieties and fears.

- Over a lifetime, 28.8 percent of those who live in the United States will suffer from one serious form of anxiety or another (Kessler et al. 2005). The numbers of people who suffer from anxieties and fears are also significant in other parts of the Westernized world (Baumeister and Härter 2007).

- Anxiety is a common worldwide debility that cuts across national, racial, and economic boundaries. Studies of people with anxiety from Qatar, Turkey, Nepal, Chili, sub-Saharan Africa, Morocco, China, and other nations contribute to this conclusion. Indeed, every continent has anxiety hot spots. The Arkhangelsk region of Russia, for example, is a high-stress location. Sixty-nine percent of the women living there and 32.3 percent of the men report high levels of anxiety, depression, and sleep problems (Averina et al. 2005).

- If you are female, you are at a greater risk for anxiety than if you are male (McLean et al. 2011).

- Being young is no buffer against anxiety. Anxiety is common among preadolescent children (Perou et al. 2013) and adolescents (Kessler et al. 2012). Anxiety increases in the middle years of life (Scott et al. 2008). Rosy numbers on lower levels of debilitating anxiety among the elderly may be a myth (Wolitzky-Taylor et al. 2010).

PUTTING A FACE ON ANXIETIES AND FEARS

You can profit from what others have learned while working on their anxiety problems in a group setting. Here's what John, Elaine, Larry, Joy, and Tom have been doing to conquer their anxieties and fears.

John's Panic

John was a frequent panicked visitor to his local hospital emergency room. Whenever he gasped for air and felt chest pains, he dialed 911. He believed that he was having a heart attack and was about to die. After more than twenty visits to the ER, and on the recommendation of his primary care physician, John joined a psychological treatment group. After three group sessions, John came to see his breathing difficulties and chest pains as symptoms of panic. He felt relieved to learn that most people with panic who learn to use exposure, relaxation, deep breathing, and other cognitive and behavioral methods make meaningful and durable progress (Sánchez-Meca et al. 2010). John aimed to join that club.

Elaine's Silence

Elaine was the group's silent member. She felt petrified at the thought of saying something foolish. After eight weeks of saying very little, she confessed that if the group leader and members really knew her, they'd kick her out of the group. The question, "Where is the evidence for that conclusion?" started Elaine thinking differently. She calmed down when she learned that her fear of rejection reflected her self-doubts and not the views of the other group members. Based on group feedback, she figured out that what she'd thought others were thinking about her could not possibly be true. The group did not necessarily have the same impressions of her that she had about herself.

Larry's Stress

Larry told the group that he became stressed easily. Like John, he had moments of panic where he had trouble breathing, he felt dizzy, and his heart beat like crazy. He said that this panic occurred when he was "stuck in one place with a lot of people in a small area." Larry went on to say that he had bad headaches. He was afraid that he might have a brain tumor.

Larry wanted to deal with his problems, but as soon as he would begin to address one anxiety or fear, he would move on to another problem without resolving the first one. He was in a revolving-door pattern of procrastination. Because his problems kept returning, he felt overwhelmed. He said, "This is too much for me to handle." His *too much* was part of an internal monologue in which he exaggerated the fearsomeness of his tensions. At the same time, Larry minimized his abilities to cope. Once he began to deal with one fear at a time, however, he found he was able to whittle down the number of his anxieties and fears. He began to feel like an emotionally freer human being.

Joy's Apprehension

Joy felt anything but joyful. She told the group that she was a dimwit in a brightly lit world of intelligent people. She argued that she made many mistakes. She dreaded the thought that people would catch on to her and discover that she was a fake.

Joy was finishing her second year of graduate school. She reported that she compulsively studied until she thought she'd have a reasonable chance of succeeding. She said, "It takes me three times as long as anyone else to pass the courses." She went silent when John asked, "How do you know how much time others spend studying? Did you take a survey?"

Although Joy received praise from her professors for the quality of her work, she claimed that she had fooled them all. The question "How can someone who sees herself as a dimwit fool others whom she sees as bright lights?" stumped her. Then Elaine pointed out that the main reason Joy felt like a dimwit was because she held a dimmer switch and turned down her own light. Joy said, "I never thought that way before." With a changing self-view, she was in a better position to celebrate her achievements. She no longer felt like a fraud.

Tom's Complacency

Tom believed that he was productive only because his fears drove him to perform. Without them, he'd be complacent. Tom feared complacency.

Tom hated being driven by his fears, but if he eased up, he believed that he would fail, and he couldn't stand failing. Tom's all-or-nothing thinking about the driving force of fear meant that he was controlled by either fear or complacency. He began to rethink this position when he was asked, "What lies in between the extremes?"

John, Elaine, Larry, Joy, and Tom participated in a supportive group where they felt free to explore their thinking, feelings, behaviors, and relationships with each other. This atmosphere promoted conditions for positive change. The following section will help you explore how to take a similarly supportive approach with yourself.

TAKING A NO-BLAME APPROACH

We live in a blame culture where we've gone overboard with blaming and defending ourselves against blame. Daily you'll see many examples of denial, rationalizations, and defensive finger pointing—all to mitigate blame. Indeed, blame is so much a part of your anxiety that you may take it for granted and ignore it. That's a mistake. Anxiety over blame cuts across most forms of needless human distress, but this huge transdiagnostic factor is rarely addressed.

By taking a no-blame approach, you may feel more inclined to experiment with new ways of thinking, feeling, and behaving. Conversely, focusing on blaming yourself will get you nowhere.

How Blame Functions

Technically, blame is a means of assigning accountability. By being accountable, or taking responsibility for correcting your anxiety problems, you are more likely to experiment with solutions. However, as you might suspect, blame is typically bloated with negative meaning, which can make it counterproductive.

More specifically, blame often comes in the form of blame *excesses* (complaining, nit-picking, faultfinding), blame *extensions* (downing and damning), and blame *exonerations* (denials, excuses, and shifting the blame), all of which are problematic. Of these, extensions of blame are especially destructive. Here is a typical process: you condemn yourself for any real or imagined faults, degrade yourself for the error, and punish yourself (in thoughts and actions) for infractions. Left unaddressed, extensions of blame thinking are a major impediment to positive change.

How Self-Acceptance Works

You can address extensions of blame thinking with self-acceptance. Self-acceptance trumps anxieties over blame. Because of a long history of living in a blame culture, however, acceptance of your inevitable mistakes may be challenging to attain and to maintain. Is it worth the effort to try? Definitely yes! A kindly, unconditional, empathic, self-accepting attitude helps mute anxiety about blame.

How might you break the connection between blame and anxiety? First, use blame strictly as a means of establishing accountability. Hold others responsible for damages that they cause. Accept responsibility for your own mistakes and accidents. Then concentrate on developing greater tolerance for your errors and working to strengthen your will to take corrective actions.

Top Tip: Concentrate Your Efforts Wisely

Dr. Daniel David is the Aaron T. Beck Professor of clinical cognitive sciences at Babeş-Bolyai University in Romania and an adjunct professor at Mount Sinai School of Medicine in New York. He is the lead editor of *Rational and Irrational Beliefs in Human Functioning*. Together, David and I developed the following top tip for curbing anxieties and fears.

You can earn relief from recurring anxieties in three interactive ways: decreasing the *intensity* of your anxious feelings (feeling better), changing the *quality* of your feelings (for example, from dysfunctional anxiety to healthy concern) by changing your thinking from exaggerations to realistic thinking, and taking steps to *engage* what you needlessly fear (doing and getting better).

To decrease the intensity of your anxiety:

- Use relaxation methods to counteract anxious arousal. For example, try square breathing. You breathe in for four seconds, hold your breath for four seconds, breathe out for four seconds, and hold that for four seconds. Repeat the cycle for about two minutes. (Square breathing can help decrease anxious arousal and set the stage for you to think clearly about your thinking.)

- Engage in purposeful distraction. For example, call a helpful friend for advice. Read material on how to calm down when your anxiety seems uncontrollable. These indirect methods can help you diminish anxious tension. However, if you use distractions, think about them as a prelude to switching from your normal flight reaction to taking concrete action steps to cope effectively.

To change the quality of your experience:

- Identify anxiety-evoking thoughts, and contest (restructure) them. For example, if you tell yourself, *I must do perfectly well in all that I undertake, or it is awful,* you are demanding what is implausible or impossible. Understandably, you'd feel anxious about your performances. To change the quality of your feelings from dysfunctional anxiety to healthy concern, substitute realistic thinking for the unrealistic variety. Instead of insisting that you do perfectly well, take a calmer, preferential approach. You can realistically tell yourself, *I'd strongly prefer to do well, and will prepare myself to do the best I can under the circumstances. If I do less well than I'd like, this is too bad but hardly the end of the world.*

- Prepare for the unexpected crisis by having rational mantras on your person. A wallet-sized card with rational expressions targeting anxiety about anxiety will do. If a crisis arises, pull out the card and repeat coping ideas, such as, "Anxiety is unpleasant, but I'll live through it. If life is not as I expect it to be, I can accept it as it is."

To directly engage your fears:

- By exposing yourself to a fear situation, without using your usual escape strategies, you've taken a solid step in the direction of building confidence in your ability to overcome fear. Here's an example: You're afraid of snakes. You make a commitment to go to the zoo and to observe a snake exhibit at a safe distance. Stay at that distance. At first, you may feel some anxiety. Stay with both the situation and the feeling of anxiety until you feel less anxious. Move a few steps closer each time you visit the exhibit. Eventually you'll get used to this situation, to the point that you can tolerate the discomfort.

- Explore shame-attacking exercises. Let's suppose that you dread making a mistake and feel exposed and ashamed when you believe that you've erred in public. By intentionally exposing yourself to what you fear, you can simultaneously change self-defeating avoidance and escapist behaviors and their underlying irrational thoughts. For example, wear two different colored socks for a day. Routinely read your mantra card to remind yourself that most people won't be picking you out from the crowd based on the color of your socks. It is hardly the end of the world if someone notices.

By routinely working to improve your emotive, cognitive, and behavioral skills, you'll have less to feel anxious about, because you'll know that you have a tested way to face them.

CORE, EMPIRICAL, AND PRACTICAL LEVELS OF CHANGE

What can you do when your anxieties and fears greatly trouble you? With core, empirical, and practical interventions, you can make deep and lasting changes.

Core Interventions

At a *core level*, you deal with deeper and more personal issues that connect to unproductive patterns in your life. For example, you might stymie yourself because of core problems, such as self-doubt, equivocating, and living in dread of making a mistake. If your anxieties are connected with self-doubt, examine the personal situations where you doubt yourself and why it is you do. Which situations are anxiety related?

If you feel both anxious and depressed, look for powerlessness thinking, where you think that you are helpless to do anything differently. Just as negative feelings can influence what you think about, your thinking processes can worsen feelings of distress. If you have multiple anxieties, are they linked with beliefs that you can't cope or won't cope adequately enough? Do you worry too much, ruminate, and procrastinate when it would be wise for you to start taking corrective actions?

Empirical Interventions

At an *empirical level*, you put on your scientist's hat. Say that you believe you can never overcome your anxiety. Will recognizing and labeling this defeatist view as an *erroneous expectation* help put this problem into perspective? Often, labeling an anxious thought can give you a sense of control over it. Now, what evidence-based interventions support what you want to accomplish? Start thinking this way, and you are on an empirical path.

Practical Interventions

At a *practical level*, you use common sense techniques to produce the changes that you want to make. For example, you acquire more information about the form of anxiety—and its antidotes—that you most want to control. You keep a log of your anxious thoughts to help reveal patterns in your anxiety thinking. You test practical solutions, such as imagining an anxious thought vaporizing like a puff of steam. You exercise to relieve tension.

EXERCISE: TAKING INVENTORY OF YOUR ANXIETIES AND FEARS

Rate each statement in the column labeled "Anxiety and Fear Issues" based on how much it applies to you over the last month. If the statement does not represent how you think and feel, circle "not you." If the statement suggests somewhat how you feel, circle "somewhat like you." If the statement reflects a persistent and bothersome issue, circle "often like you."

Your Inventory of Anxiety and Fear Issues

Anxiety and Fear Issues	Rating Scale			Intervention Chapters
"I avoid situations that I should approach."	Not you	Somewhat like you	Often like you	**12**, 2, 3, 7, 10, 16, 17
"I'm afraid of rejection."	Not you	Somewhat like you	Often like you	**22**, 1, 18, 19, 21
"My problems keep piling up."	Not you	Somewhat like you	Often like you	**7**, 2, 5, 19, 23
"I worry about making mistakes and failing."	Not you	Somewhat like you	Often like you	**19**, 2, 7, 14, 21, 22
"I'm afraid of speaking in public."	Not you	Somewhat like you	Often like you	**6**, 19, 21, 22
"I feel distressed much of the time."	Not you	Somewhat like you	Often like you	**10**, 3, 13, 14, 15, 19, 23
"I make more of a bad situation than I should."	Not you	Somewhat like you	Often like you	**5**, 1, 2, 14, 15, 17, 21, 23
"I feel held back."	Not you	Somewhat like you	Often like you	**20**, 3, 4, 13
"I don't know what to do about my anxieties."	Not you	Somewhat like you	Often like you	**2**, 3, 4, 6, 11, 13, 14, 23
"My fears and phobias control my life."	Not you	Somewhat like you	Often like you	**17**, 2, 3, 12, 18
"I feel anxious about myself."	Not you	Somewhat like you	Often like you	**21**, 2, 13, 19, 22, 23
"I worry too much."	Not you	Somewhat like you	Often like you	**13**, 3, 4, 5, 12, 14, 16, 22, 24
"My life feels like one crisis after another."	Not you	Somewhat like you	Often like you	**4**, 5, 7, 13, 14, 15, 19
"I'm sensitive about how I feel."	Not you	Somewhat like you	Often like you	**15**, **16**, 14, 21, 22, 23
"I feel both anxious and depressed."	Not you	Somewhat like you	Often like you	**23**

"I'm uncomfortable about making changes."	Not you	Somewhat like you	Often like you	**14**, 6, 7, 10, 21
"My anxious thoughts won't stop."	Not you	Somewhat like you	Often like you	**11**, 2, 4, 5, 9, 10, 13
"I need to calm down."	Not you	Somewhat like you	Often like you	**9, 8**, 12, 15, 17
"I need to take better care of myself."	Not you	Somewhat like you	Often like you	**24**, 3, 4, 15
"My anxieties and fears are complicated."	Not you	Somewhat like you	Often like you	**18**, 10, 11
"My anxiety is about as bad as it gets."	Not you	Somewhat like you	Often like you	1, 3, 5, 16, 23

After taking inventory, focus your attention on the anxiety or fear issues that are most problematic for you. The numbers on the right refer to chapters in this book where you will find practical interventions for your issues; the numbers in bold refer to chapters with the most information on these topics.

You may want to make copies of this inventory for future use. You can use it again to measure your progress. Completing the inventory once a month is a good idea. The results can serve as an early warning system to prevent a recurrence of parasitic anxieties and fears.

YOUR PROGRESS REPORT

You'll find a space like this one at the end of each chapter for you to record your progress and to record information that's worth remembering:

- Key ideas in the chapter that you found useful

- Actions you can take to combat a specific anxiety

- A description of what resulted when you executed those actions

- A description of what you learned from the experience and which actions you would reapply, modify, or discard

Write down what you learned from this chapter and what actions you plan to take. Then record what resulted from taking these actions and what you've gained.

What are three key ideas that you took away from this chapter?

1.

2.

3.

What top three actions can you take to combat a specific anxiety or fear?

1.

2.

3.

What resulted when you took these actions?

1.

2.

3.

What did you gain from taking action? What would you do differently next time?

1.

2.

3.

Doing this exercise at the end of each chapter will help you concentrate on the CBT methods that work best for you. By identifying personally relevant ideas, thinking out what to do, and testing ideas through action, you are likely to get further faster in your campaign to conquer your anxieties and fears.

CHAPTER 2

Anxieties and Fears as Friends and Foes

In Greek mythology, terror and dread are the handiwork of two gods of war who are twin brothers, Phobos and Deimos. Phobos is in charge of real and present danger. He shocks the mind with terror, panic, and flight. Deimos uses apprehension to fill minds with dread for what was to come. The ancients got it right. Fear and anxiety share many common connections, but they operate in different ways (Perkins et al. 2010).

Fear is on a proximity dimension. When in proximity to what you fear, you try to escape. Anxiety is on a time dimension. You dread a future event. You take steps to avoid it. Knowing this relationship can help you decide on which strategies to use for your anxieties and what to do to quell your fears.

FEAR ON A PROXIMITY DIMENSION

Through a telescope, you see a mountain lion a mile away. As the big cat is not close to you, you feel safe. Or say you see a mountain lion in a cage at a zoo. The cat is in close proximity, but again you feel no fear because you are in a safe place. However, if you were to come across the cat in the wild that was crouched to spring from a ledge above you, it should evoke a strong startle-fear reaction. When danger is present, and you are vulnerable, that's the *proximity dimension*.

Your natural fears come from an ancient legacy for responding to sudden changes, escaping venomous creatures and predators, and moving away from unfriendly people. On a day-by-day basis, you'll rarely find yourself in such mortal danger. However, such events do take place: say a masked stranger follows you on a dark street and appears to be getting closer.

How close do you need to be to real danger before you react? The distance where nonverbal cues normally stop conveying threat is between thirty and ninety meters away (Stamp 2012).

However, your reactions are also a matter of perception and perspective. If you face a known danger that can strike from a great distance, the rules change.

False Fear Alarms

Most fear reactions will be false. A darting shadow proves harmless. The crackling sound in the tree is a squirrel, not a leopard. Despite many false alarms, if your fear alarm saved you from injury or death even once, it did its evolutionary job. It's like an insurance policy that you hope you won't need.

What happens if a fear alarm doesn't work? Without their innate fear for the smell of cat, mice lose an important defensive fear (Kobayakawa et al. 2007). A mouse that makes no connection between the cat's odor and danger is on the cat's menu. The next time you wish you were fearless, consider that without fear you might not be alive.

Acquiring Fears

You can develop new fears through either direct or indirect experience:

- You learn not to touch a live wire because you know it would shock you. You'll learn this lesson fast, either from direct experience or knowledge that shock is painful.

- You witness a coworker getting mangled in some machinery. Later, you flinch when in that area. This a fear caused by direct observation.

- You observe how others respond to what they see as a danger (Olsson, Nearing, and Phelps 2007). A person frantically yells, "Watch out for the snake!" You never saw a live snake before, but the yell nevertheless instills fear. Later you see a snake and flinch or panic.

- You have a direct and frightening experience. You are driving in the rain and have a skidding accident near a bridge. Later, when you are driving in the rain and approaching a bridge, you fear that your vehicle will skid out of control. You grasp the wheel tightly.

These are just a few examples of how you can develop new fears.

Transitioning from False Fears to Relief

Exposure is the standard way to overcome false fears. Exposure amounts to strategically putting yourself in close proximity to your feared situation. You can do this in a graduated way. For example, you fear riding in elevators. However, you also have a job offer that you strongly want to accept, and the office where you would be working is in a skyscraper. It's impractical to walk the stairs. So what do you do? You overcome your fear of elevators by gradually exposing yourself to being in one. You may start with entering and exiting an elevator with its doors open. You would do this several times until you no longer are afraid of being in an open elevator. The next step may be riding to the first floor. And so on. Eventually, with exposure, your fear of elevators goes away.

YOUR SURVIVAL ANXIETIES

Anxiety evolved "to prepare the individual to detect and deal with threats" (Bateson, Brilot, and Nettle 2011, 707). Anxiety is sometimes like a sixth sense about uncertainties and risks that are off in the future. If you lived in prehistoric times and you felt apprehensive about running into unknown dark caves, you had a better chance of survival than someone who had no fear of caves. When anxious, what you fear is in the future. The threat comes later. This awareness can be sufficient for you to take precautions. For example, you may be naturally apprehensive upon entering unfamiliar environments. You are alert and wary. But you can respond by taking a look around. When you do, you may realize that there's nothing to fear.

In some instances, there may be a rapid transition between sensing a danger and observing it. Either way, both reactions happen within a fraction of a second (Åsli and Flaten 2012).

What Feeds Anxious Fictions

Anxiety has two essential characteristics: aroused avoidance of a future threat and relief following avoidance. That works for avoiding deadly dangers, but it does not work when negative, repetitive, and alarmist cognitions are a painful part of the anxiety process:

- Your anxieties can come in clusters, and this makes a bad situation feel worse. For example, you dread the thought of failing, so you avoid situations that evoke that threat. Or you feel anxious about rejection and avoid social situations that evoke that threat. Whenever you avoid what you dread, you reinforce avoidance so that your anxieties keep coming back.

- You dwell on your anxieties, and they grow bigger. You try to shut down your anxious thoughts, and they keep coming back. You try to subdue the feeling, and you just get more.

By correcting faulty thinking, you can decrease anxiety complications that come about as a result of it:

- False assumptions. You live in dread of something horrible happening. You're not sure what will happen, but you assume it will be catastrophic. You can learn to reverse alarmist assumptions, however. Try asking yourself, *What is the best possible scenario?*

■ Faulty expectations. You act as if you believe that the disasters that you expect to happen will inevitably happen exactly as you expect. As an alternative, you can create hypotheses that contradict the inevitability of your prediction.

■ Magnification. You dramatize every possible danger. As an alternative, magnify every bit of information that suggests the opposite conclusion. Then ask yourself, *What lies in between these magnified extremes?*

■ Possibility thinking. You make a magical jump from the possible to the probable. It's possible that your tension headache means that you have a brain tumor. To counter this thinking, ask yourself if you get this type of headache when you feel stressed. If so, what's a more logical explanation for the headache you're having?

■ Powerlessness thinking. You believe that you can't change because you are helpless. This thinking is not only pessimistic but also a formula for giving up before you start. To break this destructive pattern, act as if your mind were free of such negative thoughts. If so, what would you do? Then, take the first step.

■ Emotional reasoning. You ignore facts and ruminate on how nervous you feel. You act as if your anxious emotions verified your negative thinking and as if your negative thinking verified your anxious emotions. To get away from this circular reasoning trap, consider how a scientist would separate facts from fiction and then execute solutions that are plausible or factual. This question aids this scientific process: Where does the evidence lie?

■ Fear of the feeling. You dread feeling frustrated, uncomfortable, or afraid. You go out of your way to avoid tension, but this has a boomerang effect: you feel frustrated, uncomfortable, or afraid anyway. Allow yourself to live with the tension until you can see for yourself that these feelings can change for the better.

■ Loss of perspective. You focus on the worst-case scenario and ignore possible positive alternatives. To give yourself a new perspective, imagine an equally powerful positive scenario or result.

■ False associations. You know that home invasions are dangerous. You hear a creaking sound in your abode. You panic at the thought that someone has entered your home and intends to harm you. To counter this thought, you can ask yourself, *Does a creaking sound invariably prove that a home invasion is underway?* Do you then find yourself in a better position to judge what is actually going on?

For every anxiety-provoking thought, there is an available alternative that can decrease your feelings of anxiety.

Moving from Anxiety to Relief

Using *proactive coping*, you can work out a problem before your next anxious episode. Say, for example, that you make repeat visits to your physician with unexplained symptoms. You have headaches, gastrointestinal stress, and trouble falling asleep. You're sure you have a fatal disease. Despite test after test, you keep getting clean bills of health. You continue to ruminate about your health, but you are beginning to suspect that your dread of having an undiagnosed but fatal disease is unrealistic and exaggerated. How can you break this cycle?

You could do a reality checkup. It's true that from time to time, you will have legitimate illnesses; the problem is with worrying about a nonexistent fatal disease. Therefore, using the past six months as your time period, you would estimate the number of times you've worried about having an undiagnosed fatal disease, such as panicking over a stomachache after thinking that your stomachache means you have cancer. Perhaps you estimate that you've worried that way about a hundred times. Now over the same time period, you would look at how many times you've actually been diagnosed with an illness. You realize that you've received one diagnosis, and it was for the flu. What does that tell you?

By taking a proactive approach, you put yourself in a better position to judge when it is important to visit your physician and when it's better to eliminate exaggerations in your thinking.

YOUR SURVIVAL CIRCUITS

The mind is a part of a whole body system: "a two-way communication between the brain and the cardiovascular, immune, and other systems via neural and endocrine mechanisms. Stress is a condition of the mind-body interaction" (McEwen 2006, 367). At the core of this whole body system is a complex *survival circuit* involving cognitions, motivations, sensory systems, innate responses, learned behaviors, and other mechanisms geared toward taking advantage of opportunities, meeting challenges, thriving, and surviving (LeDoux 2012). It's a marvelous system. But what if you have excessive anxieties and fears that detract from thriving? It's useful to know what is going on.

The Amygdala

Your sensory system transmits threat information directly to your *amygdala*. This almond-shaped area of your brain is a center for fear and for some forms of anxiety (Debiec and LeDoux 2009). Your amygdala has a simple mission: avoid harm. When it comes to danger, the amygdala represents your reptile brain. Shadowing your senses, the amygdala alerts you to danger.

Your amygdala doesn't wait for a complete picture to develop before it excites stress hormones. You automatically freeze when in an enclosed place where you can't retreat. (In prehistoric times, freezing was the best survival tactic, because predators pay attention to movement.) You are super-charged to flee when that response gives you your best chance.

The amygdala is capable of learning new fears. If you were ever assaulted, for example, you might later feel tense when in an environment that reminds you of the assault.

The amygdala contributes to negative feelings by increasing your perceptual sensitivity for negative stimuli (Barrett et al. 2007). If you have a sensitive amygdala, you'll have lots of false alarms. You are more likely to overreact to things when they are not where you expect them to be, as well as to strange sounds, quick movements, or unexpected changes in emotions. In prehistoric times, those who were most sensitive to changes in their environment and sounded the alarm may have aided the survival of the group.

The Anterior Cingulate Cortex

The *anterior cingulate cortex* is a collar-shaped brain region that is located in the front part of the brain. It regulates both emotional and cognitive processes, resolves conflict between competing areas, and corrects errors. Along with your prefrontal cortex, this brain region can signal the amygdala to stop freezing or bolting.

The anterior cingulate cortex resolves conflict through corrective experiences (Posner and Rothbart 2007). It learns through comparative experience and can switch on and block the amygdala. For example, intentionally facing fictional dangers can help correct errors in perception, and neuroimaging studies illustrate that such exposure influences the prefrontal cortex, anterior cingulate cortex, and medial orbitofrontal cortex. These regions are involved in the evaluation of situations that evoke emotions, such as being near a spider when you are fearful of spiders (Linares et al. 2012).

When facing a feared situation leads to relief, neural imaging shows decreased activity in the amygdala and increased activity in the anterior cingulate cortex (Goossens et al. 2007). However, we still have much to learn about how the brain changes in response to interventions for reducing anxieties and stresses (Nechvatal and Lyons 2013).

SEPARATING REAL FROM IMAGINARY THREATS

Real anxieties and fears can coexist with misguiding anxieties and fears, and it's important to separate real from imaginary threats so that you can respond to each appropriately. This chart uses work bullying as an example of a problem that can produce both real anxieties and fears and imaginary or exaggerated ones. It suggests how you might respond in each case. (Note that the antidotes for anxiety and fear are the same when the problem is real.)

Problems and Responses	Anxiety	Fear
Real problem	You have a coworker who bullies you. After each day of work, you feel anxious about returning to work.	A coworker bullies you. You feel fear when this occurs.
How to respond	Here are some actions you could take: (1) Develop assertive communication skills to counteract the threat. (2) Ask your supervisor to intervene; perhaps management will relocate the bully. (3) Request a transfer to a different department. (4) Make a legal claim of harassment.	Here are some actions you could take: (1) Develop assertive communication skills to counteract the threat. (2) Ask your supervisor to intervene; perhaps management will relocate the bully. (3) Request a transfer to a different department. (4) Make a legal claim of harassment.
Imagined or exaggerated problem	You doubt your skill in defending your opinions and feel anxious at the thought of asserting your views.	You hold some opinions that differ from the bullying individual's opinions, but to avoid conflict, you freeze and say nothing.
How to respond	Identify the basis for your self-doubts. Examine them. Separate skill issues from fictional issues, such as the irrational need to be perfect and to make only unassailable statements. In the world of opinions, perfection is an impossible dream. Accept that sometimes you'll get agreement, and sometimes you won't, and sometimes you'll get a response where someone partially agrees and partially disagrees.	Fearsome beliefs and imaginary dreads can trigger parasitic fear alarms. You can deal with them by counteracting your parasitic thoughts and by prudently engaging in fear-related behaviors. For example, you could make a point to express at least one opinion in a discussion where others are expressing theirs. Then reflect on what you've learned. Try again, perhaps in a different way. Keep practicing until you habituate to the situation; no longer freeze when you have something that you want to say; feel confident in your views; and show adaptability, where you modify your opinions based on facts and logic.

Context is important. If the bully is your employer's mate or best friend, and you want to keep your job, some of the above solutions may not work well. Other solutions would work regardless.

EXERCISE: SEPARATING NATURAL FROM INVENTED THREATS

It's your turn. When you have a mixed natural and parasitic anxiety/fear condition, map it out. Fill in the blanks with your natural anxieties and fears, the appropriate responses, your imagined or invented anxieties and fears, and the appropriate responses.

Problems and Responses	Anxiety	Fear
Real problem		
How to respond		
Imagined or invented problem		
How to respond		

Mapping out these different emotions can be useful in helping you recognize whether real or invented emotional stresses are operating and how you can respond to each.

Top Tip: Addressing Real and Imagined Anxieties and Fears

Seton Hall University emeritus professor Dr. Jack Shannon offers his top tip for addressing a combination of natural and imaginary anxieties and fears.

"You have reason to feel concerned about an upcoming event. Your physician refers you to a surgeon who tells you that you need an operation. The operation has an 80 percent success rate. You have a 99 percent chance of dying if you do nothing. The operation is obviously necessary.

"The surgeon schedules an emergency operation in three days. Meanwhile, all you can think about is the 20 percent risk. Your anxiety level is discombobulating. You can't think clearly. Now you have a legitimate concern and an emotionally explosive parasitic view that dominates how you think and feel. But by using the following analytical approach, you can learn how to differentiate between the two states of mind and how to shift from alarmist parasitic thinking to a reasoned perspective and honest feeling of concern:

- You are understandably concerned, but you don't need to feel as if you had a 100 percent chance of dying during the operation. Can you reframe this view?

- Your parasitic option is repeatedly to remind yourself that you have a 20 percent chance of dying. Make a cognitive shift. You have an 80 percent chance for survival. Is it possible for you to magnify the 80 percent figure?

- Instead of ruminating about a worst-case scenario, use a wager technique. If you had an 80 percent chance of winning a bet, would you make a modest wager for or against your survival?

- Avoid accepting only a negative conclusion. Balance things out. Start thinking of scenarios with positive outcomes. For every negative outcome, have a positive alternative."

YOUR PROGRESS REPORT

Write down what you learned from this chapter and what actions you plan to take. Then record what resulted from taking these actions and what you've gained.

What are three key ideas that you took away from this chapter?

1.

2.

3.

What top three actions can you take to combat a specific anxiety or fear?

1.

2.

3.

What resulted when you took these actions?

1.

2.

3.

What did you gain from taking action? What would you do differently next time?

1.

2.

3.

Your Anxiety Solution

The worst kinds of anxieties and fears are the ones that you create for yourself. Fortunately, you have a powerful four-pronged solution:

1. Learn to recognize and defuse different forms of anxious thoughts and beliefs.

2. Build emotional tolerance.

3. Behaviorally engage your parasitic fears with functional new behaviors.

4. Gain mastery over yourself.

This chapter will continue the process of exploring these cognitive, emotive, and behavioral ways to execute the anxiety solution. These issues will be expanded on throughout this book.

DEFUSING ANXIETY THINKING

What-if-thinking is a form of anxiety thinking: *What if I spoke in front of a group and made a fool of myself?* or *My friend is late for our meeting. What if he was killed in an auto accident?* This form of anxious rumination is a common transdiagnostic factor. By nipping this thinking in the bud, you can eliminate considerable mental misery.

What-If-Thinking Review

You may worry: *What if an undetected asteroid threatened life on earth?* You fret about this possibility as if it were a certainty. It takes effort to break this habit of mind, but you can gain relief by accepting that you could be wrong.

First, you'd wisely recognize that this form of what-if-thinking contains erroneous information. If you believe that because the world could end in your lifetime, it will end, think again. By looking at the probabilities (not possibilities), you can reduce the uncertainty, helplessness, and vulnerability that accompanies worrying about remote possibilities. For example, what are the odds that the world will come to an end in the next year? Accept only those probability estimates that fit with known scientific facts.

Contesting Your Conclusions

Dire predictions commonly weave through worrisome what-ifs, such as *What if I got lost?* Asking a different question may help put such matters into perspective: *What am I responsible for doing when it comes to finding my way?* Obviously, you can get a map or a GPS, but that practical solution may not get to the heart of the matter.

What if your question implies that you can't count on yourself to prevent a problem or to cope with one that arises? Here's an example: *What if I appear anxious during the political rally?* Here's the implied conclusion: *People will reject me.* Now you have a core issue to explore.

To contest this core conclusion, you can ask yourself, *Where's the evidence that people at the political rally will reject me because I think that they think that I look anxious?* An honest answer would be this: *I don't precisely know what goes on in the minds of people in a crowd.* Empirical interventions like this one can help put what-if propositions into a healthy perspective.

BUILDING EMOTIONAL TOLERANCE

Emotions can whip up thoughts about themselves. You wake up in a foul mood and blame others for this feeling. Sensations of anxiety can evoke misguiding thoughts to explain the feelings, which can in turn create more anxiety. When emotions and thoughts play off each other in this way, it can be a vicious cycle.

How to Break the Cycle

What can you do if anxious thoughts and feelings feed off each other and keep you from taking action? You can start by working at developing tolerance for unpleasant feelings; you will be less likely to dread what you know you can tolerate.

Building emotional tolerance for parasitic anxieties and fears means allowing yourself to experience them. This proposition may sound unattractive. However, your willingness to endure unpleasant moods, sensations, and emotions is a tested way to boost tolerance of uncomfortable emotions. It is also a way to move in the direction of self-mastery.

Top Tip: Stop Running Away

Dr. William Golden is a faculty member at Cornell Medical College, runs an active self-help website (http://www.williamgoldenphd.com), and practices psychotherapy in New York City and in Briarcliff Manor, New York. He shares this tip on facing exaggerated threats:

"Threat and danger can be real and external, such as fire, flood, disease, or terrorists. However, the danger can be magnified, such as a fear of flying in an airplane or a fear of getting AIDS from using a public bathroom. The threat can also be from within, such as a perceived threat to your self-esteem as a result of a failure.

"Avoidance is an attempt to run away from the threat or danger. The problem with avoidance is that while giving temporary relief, it only makes matters worse in the long run, especially if the threat is based on misinformation or irrationality. In order to overcome anxiety, you need to face it both in thought and action.

"A good way to start to work on your fears and worries is to identify them. Worry is usually in the form of *What if?* An example of worry would be *What if I lose my job?* Fear, on the other hand, tends to be more specific. An example of fear would be *I'll lose my job and become homeless.* One way of dealing with fear and worry is through a reality check. Question the fear or worry: *Is there any evidence that I am going to lose my job? What is the probability that I'll lose my job?* You also can question the threat to your self-esteem. You don't become worthless as a result of losing your job. You can feel worthless only if you believe you are worthless. You can question the logic of your thinking: would you view your best friend as worthless if he or she became unemployed?

"If you still believe that there is some reality to your anxieties and fears, proceed with this five-step problem-solving approach:

1. Define the problem: In this example, "What do I do if I lose my job?"

2. Brainstorm possible solutions: For example, "I could start looking for a job now. I could start working on my resume. I could start to network. I could start an online business. I could talk to a recruiter now. I could go for career counseling. I could collect unemployment. I could negotiate a termination package."

3. Evaluate the pros and cons of each alternative. Think about the advantages and disadvantages of each option, the possible consequences to yourself and to significant others, and the possible outcomes, as well as the likelihood of success of each alternative.

4. Select the best alternative or the best combination of alternatives: you don't have to select only one option. Frequently a combination of approaches will yield the best results.

5. Implement the action plan that you have developed. If unsuccessful, instead of giving up, renew your problem solving by starting to redefine the problem, and brainstorm again. You probably will have new information and may be able to identify some new alternatives. Don't be afraid to ask other people you know and trust for their ideas. Sometimes another person can see an alternative that you missed."

How to Accept Reality

Anxiety over discomfort may be among the worst of human emotional experiences, but it can be remedied. Here are four thoughts that will help:

Discomfort won't kill you.

Unpleasant emotions eventually go away.

The only thing that feels overwhelming is the amplification of your anxious feelings.

By quelling scary ideas about tension, you'll have more time to manage the ordinary and the extraordinary stresses of life.

Emotional tolerance starts with accepting reality. If you're tense, you're tense. That's it! This does not mean capitulation to anxiety, nor does it mean that it's okay to be complacent about ruminating over what pains you.

When you dwell on discomfort, you magnify feelings that you don't want to experience and you are likely to rehash the conditions you associate with these feelings. This rehashing (negative repetitive thinking) accelerates your misery. It cuts across different forms of anxiety and other unpleasant emotional states, such as depression (McEvoy et al. 2013). If you break a rumination pattern in one area, you may automatically reduce it in another.

Although unpleasant anxious sensations sometimes do go away on their own, dwelling on a threatening situation usually makes the feelings more intense. If you no longer fear the sensations of discomfort associated with terrifying beliefs, you will be less likely to magnify them. If you don't magnify them, you'll experience less stress.

With this new level of emotional tolerance, you can begin to approach situations that trigger your anxieties and fears, which will bring about a deeper change in how you think and feel.

ENGAGING THE PROBLEM

Say you are an artist and are anxious that people will criticize and reject your sketches. Because of your fear of criticism, you ordinarily hide your work from sight. You know this is a silly fear. A number of your teachers and acquaintances have praised your talent and your sketches. You've won awards for your work. However, you once received a nasty criticism from a fellow artist, and you so dread that this will happen again that you avoid showing your work. As long as you avoid showing your work, you avoid the anxiety and fear over showing it, but you also fail to get over that anxiety and fear.

Exposure in Two Phases

The answer is to do the opposite: to behaviorally engage what you fear with functional new behaviors. You can do this in two phases: first, mentally work out the problem in stages; then in the same sequence engage what you fear.

Phase 1 might follow in four stages:

1. You start with imagining your sketches on public display.

2. You imagine yourself as a fly on the wall listening to people's comments about your work. For every negative comment that you imagine, you balance it with a corresponding positive comment.

3. You come up with five sound reasons why people have different aesthetic preferences and may not see your work in the same way. For example, some think that Leonardo da Vinci's *Mona Lisa* looks washed out or that Mona Lisa was not beautiful enough to warrant da Vinci's efforts. Yet this work is one of the most renowned paintings of all time. Here's the message: you can't please everyone. Indeed, you can't achieve perfection, and some people won't be pleased with what you do even if your work was perfect. Instead of worrying about the other guy, do the best you can.

4. You accept the validity of a pluralistic perspective (meaning that the same situation can be seen in different ways) and accept that in the case of your sketches—which will vary in quality—you have no good realistic reason to fear negative criticism from everyone, nor should you expect universal acclaim.

In phase 2, you move from this mental rehearsal to doing a behavioral exercise:

1. Hang your favorite sketches in your residence where they will be in plain view.

2. Invite people over. If you hear a negative comment, work to accept the statement without deflating yourself. (See phase 1.)

3. Remind yourself that everyone has different aesthetic preferences and may not see your work in the same way.

4. Recognize that you have no realistic reason to fear negative criticism from everyone.

As a next step, you might enter your favorite sketch in a contest and see what happens.

A Cognitive-Emotive-Behavioral Matrix for Managing Time and Proximity

Sometimes you'll feel irrationally anxious about a situation you unrealistically fear. Eventually you'll encounter the thing you were afraid of. What might you do at the point in time when anxiety merges into fear? At this point of convergence, you can use cognitive, emotive, and behavioral interventions to better manage your anxieties and fears. A matrix of cognitive, emotive, and behavioral questions can help you consider what interventions to take before you face your fear, at the point of convergence where your anxiety and fear meet, and when you are in the situation that you fear. By taking this three-pronged approach, you can manage each phase of this process.

Dimensions	Anxiety	Point of Convergence	Fear
Cognitive	*What can I do to put the threat situation into a reasoned perspective?*	*How might I think at a point of convergence, where the fear is not fully here but is in the process of becoming?*	*As I experience the fear, what can I tell myself about the situation and the sensations, so I can defeat fear-magnetizing ideas?*
Emotive	*What can I do to tolerate the physical feelings of anxiety that I do not like?*	*What actions (thoughts, behavior) can I take to cope when anxiety blends into fear?*	*What are my options when it comes to accepting the tension of fear?*
Behavioral	*What specific behaviors can I test in advance to prepare myself to cope effectively?*	*What behavioral actions can I take to face a fear at the point of convergence, where anxiety merges into fear?*	*What behavioral actions can I take to avoid retreating and reinforcing fear?*

EXERCISE: YOUR PLAN FOR MANAGING TIME AND PROXIMITY

Using this structured writing approach, write down the particular threat that you are anxious about facing. Then, using the preceding matrix of cognitive, emotive, and behavioral questions as guidelines, fill in the blanks with interventions to combat this particular threat as you approach facing it.

Your problem issue: _____ .

Dimensions	Anxiety	Point of Convergence	Fear
Cognitive			
Emotive			
Behavioral			

Top Tip: Assemble Your Change Team

Dr. John Norcross is a Distinguished Professor of Psychology at the University of Scranton, a board-certified clinical psychologist in part-time practice, and the author of *Changeology: Five Steps to Realizing Your Goals and Resolutions*. He shares this tip:

"Battling your anxiety and fears need not be a lonely pursuit. Create a change team of positive people to assist, reward, and cheer you along the way. We work better by working together. So let's buddy up.

"Some quick tips on recruiting your change team: Ask one or two people, ideally in different settings (like home, work, school, or church). You can even recruit them from online support groups. Recruit, if you can, one person who understands anxiety and has walked the anxiety walk before; courageous models and mentors spark your commitment. Not all of your friends or family members will suit your needs, so be prepared with a polite 'No, but thank you.' Beware of those enshrined in the Helper Hall of Shame: the naysayers ('It'll never work') and the 'my wayers' (those who insist that whatever worked for them will automatically work for you).

"Specify to your team what you need (listening, support, tracking your progress) and what you don't need (judgments, lectures, negativity).

"Once you start confronting and reducing the anxiety, begin employing your change team. Here's a brief checklist to ensure you're getting the most out of your helping relationships:

- *We chat frequently, several times a week at a minimum, to keep me on track.*

- *They listen to my worries and support me.*

- *I express what I need from them, even though that proves difficult sometimes.*

- *My change team keeps a positive focus and reminds me of my progress (despite the slips).*

- *When asked, they offer change tips and specific advice.*

- *We buddy up in our respective goals and even have friendly competitions to succeed.*

- *Winning teams are honest and trusting; they offer—and I accept—constructive criticism on occasion.*

- *I have tried to return the favor by asking about their needs, supporting their changes, and balancing our conversations.*

- *We celebrate our successes together!"*

YOUR PROGRESS REPORT

Write down what you learned from this chapter and what actions you plan to take. Then record what resulted from taking these actions and what you've gained.

What are three key ideas that you took away from this chapter?

1.

2.

3.

What top three actions can you take to combat a specific anxiety or fear?

1.

2.

3.

What resulted when you took these actions?

1.

2.

3.

What did you gain from taking action? What would you do differently next time?

1.

2.

3.

CHAPTER 4

Developing Your Self-Observation Skills

Anxiety is a self-absorbing process where you come to know more and more about increasingly minute issues but little about what you can do to liberate yourself from your anxiety. Paradoxically, by learning more about what you can accomplish, you learn more about your true self. So how do you get out of a myopic rut? You practice self-observation. With a self-observant approach, you take extra steps to examine your anxieties and fears as though you were watching yourself from a distance. By tracking what happens when you go through an anxiety cycle, you can discover where to intervene to change the process.

A JOURNAL FOR DOING BETTER

Writing things out can help relieve anxiety and depression, and this practice can be especially helpful for people who are unable to access quality professional services (Stockdale 2011). There are many ways to do this, including writing expressive narratives on an anxiety topic for about fifteen minutes a day for three to four days (Pennebaker and Beall 1986). You can experiment with this approach, or you can keep a daily journal. Keeping a journal will help you gather data so that you can distinguish between objectively verifiable risks and fictional dangers.

To keep a record, you can use your mobile phone, voice recognition technology, your computer, a notepad, or index cards, among other things. Choose whatever feels most natural. You are more likely to use what works best for you.

Likewise, you may choose to organize your information in a free-flowing style or in a more structured manner. A free-flowing style might mean simply recording anxiety situations and jotting down whatever comes to mind about them. If you want to use a more structured approach, you might name the evocative event, your beliefs about the event, your emotions, and your behavioral responses.

The following chart shows how to organize journal information. The example comes from a client named Bob who persistently worried. Bob started by mapping the connection between his worry situations, threat cognitions, emotions, and behaviors.

Bob's Chart of Worry Situations, Threat Cognitions, Emotions, and Behaviors

Worry Situation	Threat Cognitions	Emotions	Behaviors
Friend overdue	*Friend got into accident and may have died, and that is horrible.*	*Worry, anxiety, fear*	*Pace floor. Call friend's cell phone. Swig down a glass of wine.*
Registered letter notice	*Something dreadful is about to happen. I'm going to be sued. The IRS wants to audit my taxes.*	*Anxiety and panic, and more worry and panic as the dreaded possibilities keep coming to mind*	*Avoid the notice. Swig down a glass of wine.*
Colleague walks by me without greeting me	*I must have done something wrong. I'm being rejected. This is awful.*	*Anxiety*	*Avoid looking at colleague. Go out of way to avoid colleague. Get back at colleague by bad-mouthing him behind his back. Drink to avoid thinking of the incident.*

These three examples were sufficient to convince Bob that he tended to jump to conclusions. He noted that he drank excessively to smother his tensions when he was worried. He definitely needed to address that problem habit. His record-keeping exercise opened his eyes to what he needed to change.

EXERCISE: YOUR CHART OF WORRY SITUATIONS AND PROCESSES

Chart your own processes by writing down some examples of situations in which you are anxious or worried, your threat cognitions (what you are thinking), your emotional reactions, and behaviors.

Worry Situation	Threat Cognitions	Emotions	Behaviors

Mapping your processes can help you get a better picture of the patterns you want to break.

Examining Alternative Hypotheses

When anxieties and fears come from threatening cognitions, one way to alter the process is to come up with *alternative hypotheses*, or more positive theories about what might be true.

Suppose you received a notice for a registered letter and had no idea what it was about. The return address is blurred. You might jump to the frightening conclusion that the letter is from a lawyer who plans to sue you. You have no evidence, but you rely on the belief.

What are some alternative hypotheses? A registered letter could be a public notice that a nearby neighbor has applied for a variance to build a garage. Perhaps you forgot to update your pet's license and are being notified. The letter could be from the executor of the estate of a long-lost relative, informing you of an unexpected inheritance.

Getting the facts to see which hypothesis, if any, is correct, is the next step. You open the letter and read it. Once you know what's happening, you are in a position to decide a course of action.

The example of the registered letter shows how to identify whether you have a problem or not. Suspending judgment until you get the facts is usually a good thing to do in areas of uncertainty where you have no clue as to what's ahead—even a long time ahead.

DEALING WITH CATASTROPHIC THINKING

Albert Ellis uses the term *catastrophizing* to describe a human tendency to blow situations out of proportion, or to turn minor threats into calamities: an increase in your heart rate means that you're having a heart attack; not being able to get a song out of your head means you are going crazy. Ellis finds this thinking common among people who suffer from persistent anxieties (Ellis 2000).

Have you ever wondered why you might catastrophize? Did you observe a family member blowing things out of proportion? Did you pick it up from watching movies? These may be contributing factors. But here's another. If you startle easily, you may be prone to catastrophize and have difficulty disengaging from negative thinking (McMillan et al. 2012). Although you cannot change a tendency to startle easily, you can teach yourself to disengage from negative thinking.

Catastrophizing goes hand in hand with *awfulizing*, which means turning a bad situation into something worse (Ellis and Harper 1997). You might use alarmist language, such as "awful" or "terrible," to describe events. In this case, your inner message is that what you are feeling is worse than bad. Think again. Awfulizing amplifies what you don't like. On the other hand, toning down your language might do you considerable good. For example, substitute "unpleasant" for "awful" and see if this makes a difference.

Think About Your Thinking

In a catastrophic state of mind, you are likely to focus on what's troubling you and to neglect examining your thinking. If you find yourself catastrophizing, a solution is to think about your thinking.

Since catastrophizing is adding surplus negative meaning to a situation, you can tone down your thinking by deleting the added meaning. A good way to do this is to start with a general statement about the current effects of your anxiety and then to ask yourself what will happen next. This "and then what?" approach will help deflate a catastrophic thinking process.

Suppose you don't pass an important test. You might tell yourself that your life is ruined. You might imagine that people who know of this failure will run from you as if you had a contagious disease. But is any of this true?

Take the general statement, "My life is ruined." If this is what you say to yourself, you can question your thinking by asking, "And then what?" You might conclude, *I'll be miserable.* And then what? *I'll likely get back to my normal life.* And then what? You might conclude, *I'll study and retake the test.* If retaking the test is the bottom line, then why not go directly to that solution and bypass the catastrophic part of the process?

DEALING WITH RUMINATION

You may spend time thinking about the past and what could have been, what you did wrong, and the mistakes that you made. You think about how miserable you feel and about what's wrong with you and why you can't change. You think about what's wrong with others and why they should change. You think about what's wrong with the world and why that should change. When you feel trapped in this self-absorbing monologue, you come to know more and more about what bothers you and very little about how to escape your ruminating habit. Is it possible for you to break this cycle?

Exiting the Rumination Labyrinth

Ruminative thinking is a core issue that commonly occurs with both anxiety and depression (Olatunji et al. 2013). If you find yourself in a rumination loop, you can use your self-observation skills to defuse this process.

Step back and look at your thoughts. Nonjudgmentally *observe* (what's happening), *qualify* (what's ruminative, what's not), and *quantify* (how often, how intense, how durable) your ruminative thoughts. This examination can help to moderate rumination and worry.

Rather than look at the glass as half empty, explore what's in the other half. The world of rumination is filled with *could haves*, what you could have done or said or thought. Balance it out with memories of what you did do and are pleased with.

Reflect on the problems that you face. You can help yourself by asking productive questions and seeking verifiable answers. What are the facts in this situation? What are your options? How will you go about executing your best option? By asking and answering productive questions, you are likely to be better positioned to pursue your most promising options.

Deal with the here and now. Oscillating between regretful remembrances and anticipated dreads detracts from the present moment. Right now there is no guilt, for guilt reflects the past. Right now there is no frightful event, for anxiety is about the future. If you can't think of anything else to think about, just look at the back of your hand. What you see is what is happening right now. Not too scary, is it?

BUILDING CONFIDENT COMPOSURE

By addressing your anxieties, you can gain skills in facing adversity. These skills apply to taking advantage of positive opportunities and meeting worthy challenges, such as finding a charming mate, starting a business, or standing up for your rights when someone treats you unfairly. By recognizing misguiding anxiety thinking and avoiding vacillations that lead to procrastination, you won't waste opportunities. You're building *confident composure*, which is a state of mind where you feel in charge of yourself and of the controllable events around you.

With confident composure, you recognize that you are your own boss and no one else's. You don't demand that the world change for you, and you don't need it to change. You take life and situations as they are. You drive your actions with productive intentions. As uncertainties unfold, you decide which ones merit exploring. You allow yourself to live with tensions that are a natural part of life. With this softer but stronger view, your psychological resources are more available to defuse, finesse, or directly manage your fears, anxieties, and conflicts. You are better prepared to advance your enlightened self-interest.

Employ Realistic Optimism

By acting to overcome your parasitic anxieties and fears, you can develop *realistic optimism*, which means believing that you can apply your talents to create a brighter future by addressing today's problems now. You're primed to see opportunities and to meet worthy challenges. You also know a real threat or danger when you see one. You're motivated to prevail but also to try a different way when you come to a dead end. As a realistic optimist, you know when you are up against an immovable wall or when you can do something to tip the balance in your favor.

Consider this question: Is it possible for you to productively organize, regulate, and direct your actions to address, combat, and overcome your more debilitating parasitic anxieties and fears? If you believe that you can make an effort in good faith, you are experiencing realistic optimism and are on a path to self-mastery.

Apply Your Intellect, Ingenuity, and Will

To improve your self-observation skills, you can use three powerful faculties—your intellect, your ingenuity, and your will—to neutralize your parasitic anxieties or fears. You can use your intellect to recognize and avoid danger in advance of its occurrence. Through ingenuity, you may find a novel way to survive adversity. Your will to endure can make all the difference.

Having a higher purpose for survival, such as living for your family or fulfilling an important mission in life, immensely improves your chances of survival in dangerous circumstances. Such a purpose gives you the persistence to tolerate extreme emotional discomfort. If you are clinging to a tree in a flood, your will to endure can make a big difference. However, minor stress events are far more common.

When you are beset by anxieties and fears, you do not lose your intellect, ingenuity, or will, but sometimes these precious faculties can be misused. You use your intellect to invent excuses. You find ingenious ways to duck the discomfort of fear. You will yourself to avoid your fears. Fortunately, you can teach yourself to question excuses, put up with stresses, and come up with novel ways to address your fears.

Top Tip: Let the Monkey Fend for Itself

Atlanta psychotherapist, coauthor of *Homer the Homely Hound Dog*, and sculptor Ed Garcia offers a creative way to share space with the anxiety monkey that is on your back:

"I had a client with a fear-of-flying anxiety problem. He said that it felt as if he had a monkey on his back and that, no matter how hard he tried, he couldn't shake him off. Every time he made an effort to book a flight, that monkey held on for dear life. He never did get to buy that ticket.

"I suggested that the next time he went to book a flight, he should buy two tickets. One for himself and one for the monkey. After he recovered from my suggestion, I explained that whenever a person accepts his fear and focuses on what he wants to do, in spite of how he is feeling, the anxiety tends to become manageable. What's the monkey going to do when you bring him along? Nothing! The next time he went to book a flight, he didn't buy a ticket for the monkey. He snuck him aboard."

YOUR PROGRESS REPORT

Write down what you learned from this chapter and what actions you plan to take. Then record what resulted from taking these actions and what you've gained.

What are three key ideas that you took away from this chapter?

1.

2.

3.

What top three actions can you take to combat a specific anxiety or fear?

1.

2.

3.

What resulted when you took these actions?

1.

2.

3.

What did you gain from taking action? What would you do differently next time?

1.

2.

3.

CHAPTER 5

Defusing Double Troubles

Have you ever felt like you were in a rotating door of escalating anxieties? If so, you may have *double troubles*, which is when you make two or more problems out of one.

Here's how double troubles work. You have a problem, such as new and unexplained physical symptoms. You have a legitimate cause for concern and should go see a doctor. That's bad enough. The first layer of extra troubles comes when you read too much into the symptoms and believe that you must have a dreaded disease. Then you start worrying that you are worrying too much. You blame yourself for worrying. Because you blame yourself, you become angry at yourself. You start thinking, *I've got to get rid of this feeling, I've got to get rid of this feeling,* and you can amplify the very feelings you want to avoid. As you might guess, this problem amplification can extend into catastrophizing.

RECOGNIZING DOUBLE-TROUBLE THINKING

Double troubles come in many forms, including fearing the sensations of fear, feeling helpless over feeling helpless, and panicking over the prospect of feeling panicked. Albert Ellis (2000) describes this as a secondary disturbance where you layer a problem onto a problem.

Here is a sampling of different ways that people create double troubles with their thoughts:

- *I'm killing myself with my fears.*

- *I must stop feeling anxious now.*

- *I can't stand feeling afraid anymore.*

- *This feeling is awful. I can't take it anymore.*

- *I can't change.*

- *I'm living in hell.*

- *I'm going crazy.*

BREAKING A VICIOUS DOUBLE-TROUBLE CYCLE

Double troubles usually involve two or more of the following five conditions of mind: problem magnification, overgeneralization, urgency, helplessness and resignation, and circular thinking. Although these conditions typically occur in various combinations, you can examine and address each one separately. By changing one, you can simultaneously decrease others that are connected to the same core condition.

Problem Magnification

In problem magnification, you concentrate too much on the feared situation or tension. For example, if anxiety keeps you awake, you will have multiple double troubles if you worry about feeling tired the following day, press yourself to fall asleep, and blame yourself for feeling tense and not able to sleep. You are better off accepting that if you are anxious, you are anxious. And even if you don't fall asleep, you still can have a more restful night than if you were to wallow in distressed thinking about staying awake.

Overgeneralization

An overgeneralization is where you draw too broad a conclusion. Double troubles can reflect overgeneralizations, when you tell yourself, *I can't change* or *My fears will go on forever.* If you don't have a crystal ball, then how can you know these predictions will come true?

Urgency

Double troubles have an underlying message of urgency, such as *I must stop feeling anxious now.* The intolerance for tension in the message is unmistakable. However, a clarifying question can shift your attention. Ask yourself, *What is the worst thing that could happen if I don't stop feeling tense immediately?* Among the various possible answers, here is a rational one: you'll likely feel anxious in the next minute and survive what you are surviving now.

Helplessness

Helplessness is a belief that you can't do anything about your situation. Sometimes you can't. For example, you might want to play center for a National Football League team, but you weigh only 135 pounds. On the other hand, believing that you can't change is worth a second look. Such beliefs can be altered by new information and experience. Can you think of times when you made improvements in your life?

Circular Thinking

In most double-trouble patterns, you think in circles. Here's an example: *Because I cannot change, my fears will go on forever. Because my fears will go on forever, I cannot change.* Here's another: *Anxiety feels awful, and because it feels awful, anxiety is awful.* You can step out of a double-trouble circle by looking at each double trouble as an assumption. In the first example above, "I can't change" is an assumption. So is the second circular assumption that "fears will go on forever."

Top Tip: Bring a Worry Trip to a Happy Ending

Dr. Judith Beck is the president of the Beck Institute for Cognitive Behavior Therapy, coauthor of *Cognitive Behavior Therapy*, and the author of *The Beck Diet Solution Weight Loss Workbook*. She shares this tip on how to bring a worry trip to a happy ending:

"Many people with anxiety problems have active imaginations. When they think about a feared outcome, they often see an image in their mind's eye. For example, if you think, *What if my teenager has an accident on the highway?* you may picture his car crashing through the side rail, careening down a steep slope, and crashing into a tree.

"When you feel anxious, ask yourself whether you've been picturing a negative outcome that is unlikely to occur. If so, take control of the image and change it to a more realistic one. View yourself as the director of this minimovie. Ask yourself, *How do I want to imagine this scenario ending?* For example, you could again picture your son behind the wheel but driving reasonably on the highway, getting off at the exit, and pulling into the driveway. Changing the image will decrease your anxiety."

EXERCISING YOUR REASON

Karl Popper (1962) writes that if a statement cannot be tested and *falsified* (shown to be untrue), it pays to be skeptical of it. For example, you may believe that angels dance on the heads of pins, but can you subject this belief to a test to see if it can be falsified? You can't subject it to such a test, because the statement is a fiction.

Circular reasoning in double troubles is normally easy to falsify. The statement "My anxiety will go on forever because I cannot change, and because I cannot change, my anxiety will go on forever" is a theory, not a fact. To properly test this theory, you would look for exceptions to the statement.

You would start by defining your key terms: What does "change" mean? What does "cannot" mean? What does "forever" mean? Once the key words in a circular statement are mapped, you are in a stronger position to end double-trouble circular thinking by seeing the fallacies in the extremes.

Are all forms of circular reasoning irrational? No! Some circularity can resist falsification: "I am changing in appearance as I grow older, and as I grow older, I change in appearance." Also, not all fears are fictional, such as a feeling of fear if someone threatens you with a knife.

EXERCISE: FALSIFYING YOUR DOUBLE-TROUBLE CIRCLE OF TENSION

Examine a double-trouble circular thinking loop by taking the following steps:

1. Describe your primary double-trouble circle of tension (a statement you make to yourself):
2. Identify and define the key terms in the statement:
3. Identify exaggerations that can intensify your tension: Identify exceptions to your tension magnifying belief(s):
4. Identify your overgeneralizing ideas: Identify exceptions to your overgeneralizing belief(s):
5. Describe the results of your falsification effort:

Faulty thinking is at the heart of much amplified human misery. Being able to stop and identify faulty thinking will help you avoid it.

SEVEN WAYS TO STOP FEELING DOUBLY TROUBLED

Here are seven tips for reducing needless distress and for building confident composure. As a bonus, you can give yourself points for each tip that you know already or can accept.

Accept troubling thoughts. If you can accept that extra upset grows from magnifying the significance of an event, and you believe you can find a way to squeeze the excesses from your thinking, you can give yourself a point for making progress.

Separate distress thinking from appropriate thoughts. You may blow a true tragedy out of proportion. That's where double troubles begin. Can you separate real problems from problems where you layer one misery on top of another misery? If you can make the distinction you can give yourself a point for making progress.

Hone in on cognitive triggers. What you think about an unsettling situation can trigger emotional distress. Does feeling doubly upset result from believing that you can't control events that you believe you must control? Do you fear your own feelings? If you can make the connection between doubly upsetting ideas and their amplified emotional results, you can give yourself a point for making progress.

Look for false attributions. When nothing observable or significant happens, do you normally find something to explain your inner tension? Once you identify these inventive attributions, you can use this knowledge as an early warning signal to take quick corrective actions. You can give yourself a progress point for this accomplishment.

Classify your anxiety thinking. Anxiety thinking comes in different forms, such as exaggeration and helplessness thinking. By labeling your thoughts, you may be less likely to either exaggerate or feel helpless. Give yourself a progress point if you're able to identify these unhelpful thinking processes.

Tone down the drama. You may make too much of inconveniences, such as forgetting a password. In the process of exaggerating the inconvenience, you may use more dramatic language than the situation warrants, such as "This is too much for me to bear." Instead, describe the event in concrete terms: "I don't like the frustration of losing my password, and I would prefer that this didn't happen." You can give yourself a progress point for toning down the rhetoric.

Accept the work. Although you may quickly see your pattern of anxiety, making real progress normally takes knowledge, time, and work. When you can accept this reality, you can give yourself a progress point.

How does all of this add up? Any progress you've made suggests that you're on your way toward dropping double troubles.

EXERCISE: A DAILY DOUBLE-TROUBLE CHECKUP

If you find yourself in a double-trouble trap, copy the following checklist and use it a minimum of three weeks to give yourself a daily double-trouble checkup. Use this list to check off the tips that you've acted upon.

	S	M	T	W	T	F	S
Accept troubling thoughts.							
Separate distress from appropriate thoughts.							
Hone in on cognitive triggers.							
Look for false attributions.							
Classify anxiety thinking.							
Tone down the drama.							
Accept the work.							

As you check off the items, you'll get a double reward. You will experience fewer double troubles, which is one benefit. You will also have a visual means of seeing your progress. That's a plus!

YOUR PROGRESS REPORT

Write down what you learned from this chapter and what actions you plan to take. Then record what resulted from taking these actions and what you've gained.

What are three key ideas that you took away from this chapter?

1.

2.

3.

What top three actions can you take to combat a specific anxiety or fear?

1.

2.

3.

What resulted when you took these actions?

1.

2.

3.

What did you gain from taking action? What would you do differently next time?

1.

2.

3.

CHAPTER 6

Self-Efficacy Training to Defeat Anxiety

How do successful people meet challenges and overcome adversity? Their actions express what they believe about their capabilities. This is called *self-efficacy*, or the belief that you have the power to organize, regulate, and direct your actions to achieve mastery over challenges (Bandura 1997). The importance of self-efficacy in overcoming anxiety cannot be overstated.

- Self-efficacy plays a central role in reducing anxiety (Benight and Bandura 2004).

- Persistence in using effective counter-anxiety measures is a formula for mastery over fear and for promoting higher levels of self-efficacy (Bandura 1999).

- You are more likely to create and sustain a positive new direction if you can assign the change to your own efforts rather than to medications, the fates, or luck.

- "Self-efficacy is the major determinant of behavior, however, only when proper incentives and the necessary skills are present" (Feltz 1982, 746).

You can enhance self-efficacy by gathering information, by mastering new experiences, through imitating others' effective behaviors, through persuasion, and by developing different psychological and emotional responses. As you gather new information, you learn about the mechanisms for anxiety and how to take corrective actions. Mastering new experiences means engaging your fear in a step-by-step fashion and rewarding yourself for each significant accomplishment. Observation means watching what other people do to overcome anxiety; we learn by imitation, and you may be inclined to copy what you see. You also may benefit from the persuasion of a friend. In addition to encouraging you, a friend can accompany you when you face your fear.

If you've had bad experiences in a specific situation, such as speaking up in public, you may have developed a low self-efficacy in this area. But you can develop different psychological and emotional responses, by learning new ways to interpret your experiences. For example, you can come to view overcoming a public-speaking anxiety as a challenge rather than a threat.

A STRUCTURED APPROACH FOR CONTROLLING ANXIETY AND FEAR

By acting to reduce your anxieties, you will boost your self-efficacy, which will, in turn, reduce your stress. The following structured approach works with practically any form of anxiety. It uses public-speaking anxiety as an example, since that is one of the more common forms of social anxieties. There are six phases to this self-efficacy plan: analyzing the problem, stating your mission, setting goals, planning action, executing your plan, and evaluating how you are doing.

Analyzing the Problem

Fear of public speaking is grounded in negative expectations, anxieties about being evaluated, self-consciousness, and fear of rejection. You are likely to focus on what went wrong in the past and blow that out of proportion (Cody and Teachman 2011). These negative reminiscences help keep anxiety alive.

An analysis of a public-speaking anxiety might start with examining the cognitive, emotive, and behavioral components of the anxiety. This analysis can point to where you can correct malfunctions. Here are four areas to explore as you launch a cognitive, emotive, behavioral analysis of your own fears.

What external situations are likely to activate your anxiety and fear? An external event might be a public-speech assignment, an opportunity to ask a question, or the task of making small talk at a social gathering.

What do you tell yourself about these situations that intensify your anxiety and fear? Like the Amazon River, thinking flows uninterrupted. You will practically always be thinking about something. (Try to stop thinking for the next five minutes and see what happens.) Think about your thinking. Do you hear yourself saying something like *Failure would be horrible* when you anticipate speaking?

What adds to your anxiety? Anxieties and fears rarely occur independently of other conditions, such as perfectionism, blame, procrastination, insecurity, and inhibition. For example, if you believe that you must give a perfect talk, one in which every statement is unassailable, you are living an impossible dream.

How can you develop a challenge outlook? Approaching public speaking as a challenge is remarkably different from retreating from the same situation that you define as a threat. When you gain mastery over public speaking, your heart pumps more efficiently because your blood flows with less resistance. On the other hand, a threat outlook about public speaking leads to vascular constriction. The heart pumps harder to get blood through the system (Blascovich et al. 2011). In giving speeches, students whose physiological measures were consistent with a challenge outlook got higher course grades (Seery et al. 2010).

EXERCISE: YOUR PERSONAL PROBLEM ANALYSIS

Analyze your particular anxieties and fears by answering this set of questions:

1. What external situations are likely to activate your particular anxieties and fears?
2. What do you tell yourself about these situations that evoke or intensify your anxiety and fears?
3. What coexisting conditions add to your vulnerability for distress?
4. What basic steps can you take to overcome your anxieties and also defuse coexisting conditions?
5. What can you do to give yourself a challenge outlook?

Doing this analysis gives you a way to organize your thinking around a challenge approach.

As you switch from a threat outlook to a challenge outlook, you will stop avoiding threats and begin approaching beneficial situations.

Stating Your Mission

A mission is a statement of purpose. A self-improvement mission statement expresses what you want to accomplish and how you plan to do it. Here are some examples of mission statements for overcoming anxieties and fears:

■ "I will reduce fear by challenging helplessness thinking."

■ "I will counteract fearsome images by balancing them with tranquility images."

■ "I will decrease my social fears by developing small-talk skills."

EXERCISE: STATE YOUR MISSION

What is your prime mission when it comes to overcoming your main fear or anxiety? Use this space to state your mission.

_____

_____

_____

_____

Setting Goals

To reach your mission, you need relevant, measurable, and achievable goals.

■ If your goal is relevant and consistent with an objectively positive personal and social outcome, it's probably worth stretching to achieve. Being able to speak in public is a concrete goal that is relevant if you want to stop feeling afraid of speaking up in groups.

■ If your goal is measurable, you can track your progress. Identifying and changing fear thinking about public speaking is a measurable goal.

■ Knowing that a goal is achievable can motivate you to pursue it. Progressively mastering ways to develop effective public-speaking skills is an achievable goal.

EXERCISE: NAME YOUR PRIMARY GOAL

Executing purposeful, measurable, and achievable goals is the basic path to obtaining positive results. State your primary goal:

_____

_____

Top Tip: Accept Your Public-Speaking Anxiety

Manhattan psychologist and psychotherapist Dr. Ron Murphy shares his thoughts on when admitting to a public-speaking anxiety can help you become a more relaxed speaker:

"Lots of people are needlessly ashamed that they suffer from anxiety. While it's true that not everyone experiences intense or persistent anxiety, those who do so are the end product of long evolutionary development. Millions of years of human survival have given us an exquisitely developed flight-or-fight response. As early members of our species crossed the savanna, the ones looking over their shoulders had a lot better chance of staying alive and reproducing than the ones grooving on the pretty cloud formations. So, painful anxiety is too much of a good thing, not anything shameful. It's kind of like having a Ferrari engine in a golf cart. More than we need, but better than no engine at all.

"Trying to mask or hide anxiety because we think it shameful usually makes it worse. A common example of this relates to public speaking and other social anxieties. Very often, the thought that scares us the most is that someone may notice that we are anxious! _Quelle horreur!_ If we can accept our anxiety, we can acknowledge it up front and stop wasting energy hiding it from others, which almost always backfires. Many speakers have found that starting off by mentioning their anxiety to an audience helps them relax considerably. Afterward, they are usually told their admission made them more human and likable, not weak and fearful. Try it sometime!"

Planning Action

An action plan defines the steps that you will take and the order in which you will take them. Action plans typically answer three questions: Where are you starting from? Where are you heading? What do you need to do to get there?

The answer to the first question is simple. You start with an anxiety or fear, such as a public-speaking anxiety, that you want to minimize or eliminate.

Where are you heading? If public speaking is your issue, you are ultimately heading toward speaking before groups with little more than normal apprehension or stage fright and maybe with a positive anticipation of being able to convey your ideas to the audience.

What do you need to do to get there? Your plan would naturally involve meeting objectives to fulfill goals that support your mission. For example, you'd develop cognitive skills to reduce negative forecasting; build emotional tolerance for distress; and take behavioral steps to manage, minimize, or overcome your public-speaking anxieties and fears. And you'd distinguish between what is relevant and what is unfounded in your automatic negative thoughts. People who follow this self-observant approach show significant improvement (Philippot, Vrielynck, and Muller 2010).

Recognizing Barriers

Distractions and detours are bound to get in the way of even the best-laid plans, so prepare for possible obstacles. Good plans take potential barriers into account. Thus, it's important to learn to recognize and cope with anything that could get in your way. If you know the barriers you face, you can do something about cutting through them. Here are some possibilities:

- Ambivalence. You want the change but not to experience the doubts and the tension associated with it, so you take no action. To overcome ambivalence, look for a balance-tipping idea or reason to get going on addressing your anxieties. Perhaps you want liberation from the anxiety.

- Reactance. You view taking action to change as interfering with your freedom to stay in a safe haven. To overcome this barrier, do a cost-benefit analysis. Perhaps acting to overcome anxiety competes with avoiding anxiety. But where do you get your biggest payoff, from retreating or advancing?

- Emotional reasoning, where you believe you have to feel comfortable before undertaking something uncomfortable. Overcoming anxiety is ordinarily not a comfortable process. If you can accept discomfort as part of the process, you are moving in the right direction.

Executing Your Plan

A tested way to rid yourself of a needless fear is to engage what you fear. I know that may sound like an unpleasant option. But ridding yourself of fear involves experiencing fear as part of the solution. If you have a fear of public speaking, the odds are that you will experience an unpleasant arousal once you face a public-speaking situation. A critical part of this phase involves staying with your sensations of fear until they subside. That's a feature of change that many hate to hear. However, by allowing yourself to live through the feelings that you'd ordinarily avoid, you'll have shown yourself that you can survive them. You'll likely find that your anxious feelings fade over time.

Evaluating How You Are Doing

Certain guidelines will help you gauge if you are moving forward with your self-efficacy program to overcome a public-speaking anxiety (or other situation where you experience anxiety and fear). You can ask yourself the following set of questions:

- Does your mission state a clear purpose?

- Have you set relevant goals?

- Does your plan contain sufficient details and directions to accomplish your mission?

- Have you executed your plan?

If the answer to each of these questions is yes, then you know you are moving in the right direction. If the answer to any is no, then go back and look at what may be getting in your way.

Once you execute your plan, you can continue to evaluate how you are doing. There are three classic ways to measure mastery over anxiety or fear:

- You are thinking more clearly.

- You are feeling better.

- You are seeing positive changes in your behavior.

After evaluating how you are doing, you may decide that you are on the right track, or that you need to modify your approach or try a different way.

YOUR PROGRESS REPORT

Write down what you learned from this chapter and what actions you plan to take. Then record what resulted from taking these actions and what you've gained.

What are three key ideas that you took away from this chapter?

1.

2.

3.

What top three actions can you take to combat a specific anxiety or fear?

1.

2.

3.

What resulted when you took these actions?

1.

2.

3.

What did you gain from taking action? What would you do differently next time?

1.

2.

3.

CHAPTER 7

Breaking the
Anxiety-Procrastination Connection

Procrastination is a major transdiagnostic issue that can spread like an out-of-control weed. It's a habit of missing deadlines and avoiding problems. It's a symptom of anxiety, depression, or other emotional conditions. It's a defense against facing a specific issue such as intolerance for uncertainty or fear of failure. It can include all of the above and more.

PROCRASTINATION IS A PROCESS

Procrastination is an automatic problem habit of needlessly delaying a timely, relevant, priority activity until another day or time. But to understand how procrastination works, you need to see it as a living process with specific stages.

You can break the process of procrastination down into commonly observed phases. The left column of this chart gives a sample procrastination process, with stages moving from the top down. Sample interventions for each stage are given on the right.

Sample Procrastination Process	Sample Interventions
1. Procrastination normally starts with anticipation. You face a priority activity that you initially perceive as uncomfortable. (This discomfort can be as slight as a whisper of negative affect.)	Plan to follow through even when you would normally sidetrack to safer or less timely activities.

2. You evaluate this timely activity as uncomfortable, inconvenient, threatening, tedious, boring, or frightening.	Negative evaluations about the threats or tediousness of a priority activity may be true. But it doesn't follow that you have to avoid timely and relevant activities because you don't like or want to do them. Add a countermanding comment, such as "Life has some unpleasant duties and obligations and responsibilities. I'll act responsibly whether I like the task or not, or whether I fear the task or not." (This is a position of maturity.)
3. You *always* substitute something safer, less threatening, or less timely for what you are putting off. You text a friend to ask about the weather. You read a novel. You wash your car. You feel relief from this retreat and are likely to repeat what you did to obtain relief.	Remind yourself that diversions are the *sine qua non* of procrastination. If you don't divert your attention, you'll engage your priority, which is what is in your best interest to do.
4. You'll practically always justify the delay by advancing an argument to yourself that you are too tired, too weak, too disinterested, or too anxious to follow through.	Tune in to your justifications, such as *This is too tough. I can't take the anxiety.* Label such evaluation as *exaggerations that amplify anxious emotions* and refuse to accept it as factual.
5. Procrastination practically always includes procrastination thinking. You make promises to yourself that you rarely keep: *I'll do better next time. I'll start later when I feel better. I need to let the issue season.*	Listen for procrastination thinking, such as *I'm too tired* or *I'll do this tomorrow.* Revise these procrastination decision thoughts to *I'll start something now. Then I'll judge the difficulty. Then I'll decide what I'll do next.*
6. You may feel relief (and off the hook) by making a decision to delay. This relief serves to reinforce future procrastination decisions.	Live through the discomfort as you engage the task. Your important reward comes later, when you've progressed with your self-improvement initiative; and still later, when you gain mastery over this anxiety-procrastination process.

EXERCISE: YOUR PROCRASTINATION PROCESS

Now it's your turn to map your procrastination process and decide what will work for you in the way of interventions. Fill in the stages of what you tend to do. Then write down how you can intervene at each stage to stop procrastinating at any point.

Your Procrastination Process	Your Interventions
1.	
2.	
3.	
4.	
5.	
6.	

Once you see what's happening, you can take steps to change this process and benefit from timely actions.

SECONDARY PROCRASTINATION

When procrastination is a basic habit of delay, it is known as *primary procrastination*. Scattered acts of primary procrastination may not amount to much, but patterns do! You may feel anxious and overwhelmed over a pileup of tasks that you've put off. Although primary procrastination doesn't automatically lead to anxiety, delaying often leads to feeling pressured, feeling anxious, complaining that you have too much to do, and running out of time. And of course, a pattern of delay can prove disadvantageous in other ways when you lose opportunities by letting them slide by.

When procrastination is a symptom of anxiety, it is *secondary procrastination*. The anxiety is primary. Procrastination is a symptom of anxiety.

When anxiety and procrastination coexist, you're in a cycle of misery: you automatically avoid what you fear, you put off actions to end your avoidance cycle, and you put off efforts to start overcoming the fear. Unless you take corrective action, you'll lose opportunities to self-improve. You'll repeat the cycle. Here, procrastination is an impediment to overcoming itself as well as to combatting anxiety.

Anxiety and procrastination can overlap. For example, both anxiety and procrastination may arise from self-doubts, fear of uncertainty, or a sense of lack of control.

When contending with an anxiety-procrastination connection, you have at least two challenges: combatting your initial procrastination on addressing anxiety (getting information about anxiety and applying what you learn) and combatting procrastination that shadows anxiety (failing to follow through on activities because you associate them with feeling anxious).

The next section uses anxiety over failure as an example of how to apply cognitive, emotive, and behavioral methods to break this anxiety-procrastination connection.

FEAR OF FAILURE AND SECONDARY PROCRASTINATION

What can you do if you find yourself procrastinating when anxiety about failing is the issue? This chart looks at the cognitive, emotional, and behavioral dimensions of procrastination diversions and at productive alternatives, action plans, and possible results of taking action.

Anxiety you put off facing: *Anxiety over failing an academic test.*

Dimensions	Procrastination Diversions	Productive Alternatives	Action Plan	Results
Cognitive	Tell yourself that you'll feel more relaxed and ready to study after attending a party.	Rather than divert yourself, apply the time to studying.	Accept that studying can feel frustrating and that frustration is a normal part of formal education.	Greater tolerance for frustration. Progress with studying.
Emotive	Tell yourself that you have to be in the right mood to study.	Consider the idea that motivation can follow action.	Accept that you don't need to feel inspired to do what you consider uninspiring when it is instrumental to achieving the goal of passing a test.	Proceed to study as you would approach other work tasks that involve time and concentration.
Behavioral	Attend party.	Use "party time" to study.	Announce to your friends that you intend to study.	Friends leave, allowing you to prepare for the test.

EXERCISE: YOUR ANXIETY-PROCRASTINATION CONNECTION

Use this format to break your own anxiety-procrastination connection. Fill in the blanks, first by writing down the anxiety you put off facing. Then map out your cognitive, emotive, and behavioral procrastination diversions, productive alternatives, your action plan for each, and the results of executing these plans.

Anxiety you put off facing: _____.

Dimensions	Procrastination Diversions	Productive Alternatives	Action Plan	Results
Cognitive				
Emotive				
Behavioral				

It's a paradox that a habit of avoiding work takes work to correct. Nevertheless, in the long term, this is the best way to get out of a pattern where you keep cycling through anxiety and procrastination over and over and get nowhere.

PROCRASTINATION, EMOTIONS, AND DECISION MAKING

In the prehistoric world, our ancestors thrived and survived by going for what was available, such as low-hanging fruit on a tree. Times change, but that tendency remains.

When what is immediately before your eyes looms large, you may discount the value of a later greater gain (Ainslie 2005). Sometimes this is no big deal. You sample a spoonful of ice cream when your goal is to lose weight. Impulse also can be self-defeating. It's easier to run up a big credit card debt than to save for retirement. It's more fun to party than to study for tomorrow's examination. You also have other capabilities, such as your ability to exercise foresight and resist impulse. You put away money for retirement. You study instead of going to a party.

The ancient Greek centaur myth shows the problem with going for short-term rewards while neglecting long-term important rewards because they seem too far off into the future. Half-human and half-horse, the centaur had wild animal instincts but was capable of human wisdom and reason.

Imagine you were a centaur and torn between two natures. You would face a never-ending conflict between nature and reason. The horse side of your personality would seek pleasure and avoid discomfort. When in charge, the horse heads for the field to graze, the stream to drink, and the barn to sleep. The horse's normal inclination is to follow the path of least resistance. But that may not always be the smartest path to take. Nevertheless, the horse is a powerful driving force.

Now comes Chiron, the wisest and greatest of the centaurs. He represents the best of both worlds. He has the gift of teaching and guiding. Chiron understands the importance of resisting impulsive actions and going for longer-term benefits when they are appropriate and desirable.

Like the centaur, we operate at two levels. There is a biological level that Joseph LeDoux (2012) describes as a basic survival circuit that is wired to negotiate opportunities and meet challenges in life. But we also live in a social world where a certain amount of conformity is necessary. Some of our responsibilities are to follow through on socially prescribed commitments, which includes meeting deadlines.

Thus, you will feel pushed and pulled in different directions. When it comes to fulfilling responsibilities and securing long-term benefits, asserting self-control is important. When you are caught in a tug-of-war between competing drives, perspective is important. Perhaps Chiron can help.

Solving the Double-Agenda Procrastination Dilemma

When you suffer from secondary procrastination, it's like having a double agenda. You have your stated agenda, which is to overcome a problem anxiety. You also have an implied agenda, which is to dodge discomfort. When dodging discomfort is your top priority, you'll be inclined to dwell on negative possibilities. You'll be likely to procrastinate on addressing challenges that can bring relief from anxiety. You'll be operating with an "I want relief now" view. But where does that get you?

Whenever your mind says to take time to solve a problem, and your gratification instincts pull you in the other direction, you have a Y *decision* to make, in which one branch of the Y points toward going for what is quickest and easiest and discounting future consequences. The other branch of the Y points toward restraining impulses so that you can have later, greater gains. Thus, the crux of the Y decision is whether to follow the path of least resistance or to follow the path of productive actions in which you combat and overcome what you fear.

Acting with Chiron as Your Guide

In resolving a double-agenda dilemma, you face at least two challenges. One is to recognize the conflict. The other is to apply your organizing, directing, and regulating abilities (self-efficacy) to achieve your stated goal of overcoming anxiety and achieving things in life that you put off because of anxiety.

With Chiron as your guide, you can learn that within your nature you have powerful forces to avoid threats and escape dangers. However, primitive escape and avoidance drives are sometimes misaligned in a social world where you have schedules and responsibilities. From this perspective, it doesn't matter that you want to avoid hassle and anxieties associated with legitimate responsibilities. Sometimes you'll need to override these urges when doing so is in your enlightened self-interest.

Taking Charge

Fear, anxiety, and procrastination share a common feature: an impulse to dodge discomfort. Building emotional resilience and stamina is a by-product of allowing yourself to experience discomfort as you choose to do a timely priority activity.

There are many ways to take charge. Psychologist John Dollard (1942, 22) writes, "When afraid, stop and think. Examine the feared situation. See if there is any real danger in it. If not, try just that act to which the fear is attached."

Thinking things through and acting on your analysis can be challenging to do, and you may put this off for many reasons. Here are a few examples:

■ You want to avoid stirring up unpleasant emotions. For example, you have a public-speaking anxiety, so you feel anxious when you think about giving a talk. Therefore, you avoid both thinking about speaking and thinking about overcoming your anxiety.

- You want to leave your current job and get a better one, but you procrastinate because you are afraid that you may look like a jerk during a job interview. To avoid that anxiety, you stay in a job that you hate.

- You want to avoid having to choose the lesser of two evils. You are in a relationship with a person who acts destructively, but because you are anxious about living alone, you put off thinking through and acting upon your enlightened options.

However, there are many ways to put yourself on a productive path:

Keep a procrastination log. In the log, describe your anxiety situation, procrastination thinking, and how you are feeling. Examine the contents of your procrastination log. Use this information to forge a strategy of positive change.

When a fearsome situation looms, think about your thinking. What do you tell yourself about the situation you're avoiding? What do you tell yourself about the emotions that you feel? What would Chiron say to do?

Design a self-efficacy plan for breaking an anxiety-procrastination connection. Set a mission. Establish goals. Make a plan. Organize your resources. Execute the plan. Review the results. Make revisions.

Execute an antihelplessness exercise for thinking things through. If you believe that you are helpless and therefore can do nothing to stop feeling anxious, use the *impossibility exercise*. Instead of saying, "I can't act," say, "It's impossible for me to take any action whatsoever to either do or get better." All you need is one contrary example to falsify a procrastination-provoking assumption like this one.

Do a benefits analysis. Ask yourself about the short- and long-term benefits of bolting and avoiding vs. the short- and long-term benefits of pushing yourself to meet the challenge. Does this analysis help?

Use the mnemonic EMOTION to remind yourself to follow through: **E**nergize your priority efforts by addressing the most important first. **M**ove yourself toward achieving productive outcomes. **O**perate by keeping your focus on long-term advantages. **T**olerate but don't give in to emotional signals for needless delays. **I**ntegrate realistic thinking with self-regulated actions to achieve stated objectives. **O**vercome diversionary unstated agenda urges with "do it now" actions. **N**udge yourself in the direction of Y decisions that lead to productive results.

THE PROCRASTINATION ENDGAME

The procrastination endgame involves grinding it out to produce new results by using your intelligence, ingenuity, and will to overcome a complex anxiety-procrastination connection. This strategy sets the stage for many positive outcomes:

- Strengthened ability to execute your responsibilities efficiently and effectively

- Better developed maturity through competent action

- Avoidance of needless stress and behavioral consequences that can come from excessive delay

- More free time created for pleasurable pursuits

- Advantages gained from developing a reputation as an effective person

- The self-confidence that comes from directing your actions to achieve positive results

- Tolerance for frustration as a buffer against needless distresses

By playing the procrastination endgame, you can quickly discover that unpleasant avoidance feelings ebb as you work through them. That's how to beat secondary procrastination due to anxiety.

Top Tip: Anxiety Won't Kill You

Will Ross, webmaster of REBTnetwork.org, hotline counselor, and self-help writer, offers his view on how we acquire nuisance anxieties and fears and how to rid ourselves of these distractions:

"In the early days of human history, our ability to create anxiety kept us alive; it was a survival mechanism. These days, our ability to create needless anxieties is a damn nuisance. We make ourselves anxious when (1) we perceive a threat to our comfort or well-being or to our ego; (2) we overestimate the harm the threat will cause and/or we underestimate our ability to cope with the threat; and (3) we convince ourselves that we need to avoid the threat.

"Fortunately, we have an antidote to anxiety. Just as we create our anxiety with our thoughts, we can uncreate it by thoroughly convincing ourselves that (1) whatever is threatening us isn't the end of the world; (2) we'll survive the threat—it won't kill us; and (3) we don't need to avoid it."

YOUR PROGRESS REPORT

Write down what you learned from this chapter and what actions you plan to take. Then record what resulted from taking these actions and what you've gained.

What are three key ideas that you took away from this chapter?

1.

2.

3.

What top three actions can you take to combat a specific anxiety or fear?

1.

2.

3.

What resulted when you took these actions?

1.

2.

3.

What did you gain from taking action? What would you do differently next time?

1.

2.

3.

PART II

Cognitive, Emotive, and Behavioral Ways to Defeat Anxiety

- Use natural scenes to calm your mind.

- Create tranquil feelings with music.

- Activate yourself and approach opportunities you'd ordinarily avoid because of anxiety.

- Use proven ways to relax your body and mind.

- Stop thinking yourself into an emotional tizzy.

- Apply a reversal technique and use your imagination to contain anxiety.

- Control your anxieties and fears with a special five-step metacognitive plan.

- Discover how to stop thinking in circles about your anxieties and fears.

- Learn how to use an ABCDE method to overcome your anxieties and fears.

- Follow a time-and-proximity system to combat specific fears.

- Use a simple card-sort method to organize a campaign against fear.

- Address emotional trauma in an organized way.

CHAPTER 8

Scenes for Serenity

Practically everybody has a favorite natural landscape that they associate with tranquility. You may appreciate ocean waves along a beach or a sunset over a distant mountain. By viewing scenes that you associate with thriving and surviving, you can create a tranquil effect within yourself. This chapter offers a number of methods for incorporating scenic views into your daily life: from looking at photographs of beautiful landscapes to getting exercise on a nature walk to enjoying scenes of serenity while listening to relaxing music.

EVOKING TRANQUILITY

For many reasons, being out in nature or simply viewing a nature scene can have a calming effect. What landscapes you choose to view can influence the type of mood or emotion that you want to produce (Sabatinelli et al. 2011). Tranquil scenes connect you to an ancient calling for safe, secure, pleasant habitats. Green areas with water seem to have strong positive impact (Barton and Pretty 2010). Clear water scenes are highly desired and include mountain waterfalls, oceans, rivers, lakes, and ponds (McAndrew et al. 1998). Receding paths and rivers appeal to our curiosity, interest in mystery, and sense of fascination (Dutton 2003). Open spaces may be more important than places (Kravitz, Peng, and Baker 2011). A combination of openness and complexity (a scene that includes a stream) can trigger an urge to explore. Out-of-place objects can be distracting (Walther et al. 2009). If you observe a beautiful natural landscape cluttered by beer cans, you may feel disgusted. Dark shadows that seem foreboding can disrupt the tranquility of a scene. Nature gets the edge over viewing human-built structures (Ulrich 1977). However, looking out at open scenes from human-made structures is a preferred vantage point (Stamps 2008).

Being out in nature can have a calming effect on the nervous system. Five minutes of exercise in a park, working in a garden, kayaking, or walking a nature trail can be relaxing if you have been feeling stressed. But simply viewing a photograph or a painting of a nature scene can also have a calming effect. Experiment. Discover what works best for you.

Aesthetic and pleasing nature scenes can reduce feelings of stress and promote well-being (Velarde, Fry, and Tveit 2007). In comparing nature to urban scenes, exposure to nature paintings in office settings decreases stress and anger (Kweon et al. 2008). Nature scenes are associated with a faster recovery from stress than urban scenes are (Brown, Barton, and Gladwell 2013). For those living in poverty areas, viewing open green environments is associated with reduced mental fatigue (Kuo 2001). Interestingly, tranquility scenes are relatively constant across places and cultures. Variations are based in region and enculturation (Falk and Balling 2010).

Top Tip: Restraining Anxiety with Relaxation and Reason

Dr. Irwin Altrows is a training supervisor in rational emotive behavior therapy, and an adjunct assistant professor (psychiatry and psychology) at Queen's University, Kingston, Canada. He shares this tip with you:

"Even in a state of high anxiety, your mind is capable of holding on to reason and gaining control, like a pilot landing a plane in the midst of turbulence. Next time you feel overwhelmed by anxiety, here is an experiment to try. For best results, first practice in calm moments many times: imagine a moderately difficult problem, do the first step using scenes and words that are relaxing for you personally, and follow through with the remaining steps. Then if you feel overwhelmed by anxiety in a real situation, carry out these five simple steps:

1. Conjure a peaceful image. Picture a blue lake with a warm breeze flowing over the waters creating ripples that glisten in the sun. Imagine the sound of waves lapping onto the shore. Now think the words 'calm, peaceful, serene.'

2. Observe your success. Because you can imagine the lake, breeze, ripples, and sounds and you can think the words 'calm, peaceful, serene,' you are not locked into your anxious line of thought.

3. Consider what action you might take to successfully resolve your anxious situation.

4. Picture yourself calmly taking the first step.

5. Take it!

LANDSCAPE VIEWS AND YOU

You may enjoy looking at a waterfall or seeing a wheat field beside a country road. These scenes can temporarily boost your memory, heighten attention, and improve your performance on cognitive tasks (Berman, Jonides, and Kaplan 2008).What if you live in a populated area where natural scenes are not readily available? If you have a preferred nature scene that you can see from a window, make a point of looking outside each day. If you are surrounded by concrete or wooden structures and there are no open green spaces, put pleasing-looking plants on your windowsill.

Combining Nature Scenes with Exercise

By viewing pleasant nature scenery and getting physical exercise at the same time, you may gain more than you would by doing either alone. Exercising outdoors appears to have a quicker positive effect on mood and well-being than working out in a social club or gym (Barton, Griffin, and Pretty 2012).

EXERCISE: WALKING IN NATURE

Take a daily walk outdoors for a half hour or longer, going through areas with pleasing natural visual scenery, such as by a river or by a stream with open vistas. If you are in a metropolitan setting, you can go on walking or biking trails, or to parks that are known for their outdoor spaces. A large public park with grassy areas, walking trails, and water might do. If you are traveling to a large metropolitan area, you can do a general web search for "trails near [city]."

Exercise in itself is a good way to relieve tension. Getting exercise in a beautiful space outdoors can be even more beneficial.

Tranquility and Landscape Picture Scenes

If you don't have immediate access to nature, landscape photographs can be a good substitute (Stamps 2010). Looking at photos of nature scenery can have a calming effect and improve your ability to attend to and focus on cognitive tasks. Landscape paintings, photos, and imagery-rich verbal descriptions of tranquil scenes can evoke tranquil feelings (Dunn 1976). Scenic color photos can evoke the same feelings as being in nature (Stamps 1990).

There are many ways to use photo images to help promote relaxation:

- A classic tranquil scene is an open space with trees and a river and a mountain range in the background. Select photo scenes with open spaces that suggest a clear line of sight.

- Pay attention to color. Your world is surrounded by blue skies and green landscapes. It's not surprising that blue and green are common favorite colors that are associated with tranquility. Select scenes with natural blue and green colors.

- Use landscape scenes as wallpaper on your computer screen; pick scenes that you associate with tranquility.

- Decorate your work area at home or at your workplace with tranquil landscape scenes. Place them prominently, where you can frequently see them.

- Practice visualizing landscape scenes that appeal to you. Visualizing such scenes can have a calming effect.

By looking at natural scenery on a daily basis, you may have pleasing experiences that accumulate over time. Although there is no longitudinal research on the long-term effects of experiencing open landscape scenes, it's noteworthy that people pay premiums for living in scenic areas.

APPROACHING OPPORTUNITIES

If you feel anxious about an approaching opportunity and want to motivate yourself, try repeating activating phrases while imagining or looking at views of calming nature scenery, then launch yourself into the activity.

EXERCISE: RELAX AND ACTIVATE

Take these steps to relax and to get motivated to pursue a meaningful goal.

1. Start with a meaningful goal that relates to thriving, such as studying for an important test, which you are putting off because you feel apprehensive.

2. Decide on the first step that you will take, such as opening a book to study.

3. Select a visual image that evokes tranquility, such as your favorite ocean scene.

4. Come up with three activating phrases that give directions for achieving your goal. Examples would be "I have passing the test in mind," "I feel relaxed and ready to act," or "I'm opening the book to study."

5. Think about or look at a picture of the visual image that you chose in step 3 until you feel tranquil.

6. Keep the tranquil image in mind and repeat each of your activating phrases six times.

7. Launch action by opening the book.

Top Tip: Five Phases of Photographing Landscape Scenes

Dale Jarvis of Fayetteville, North Carolina—graphics designer, professional photographer, and AreaOne Art and Design president—shares five tips for photographing tranquility-evoking landscape scenes:

"Follow the six Ps that professional photographers follow: Prior proper planning prevents poor photography.

"Ask yourself, *What do I want to see in the shot?* Keep this question in mind as you sight what you want to shoot. This phase of your composition will largely determine what you are likely to get.

"All photos have width and height. Interest in the photo scene increases with depth. Be mindful of the foreground, middle ground, and background. That can help create a sense of depth.

"Make good use of a foreground object. If possible, place a flower or tree or another object close to the camera to add interest and depth.

"When possible, use the golden hour for your natural landscape photos. The hour is thirty minutes before and thirty minutes after sunrise and sunset. Conditions are most favorable at that time for creating a quality photo image."

MUSIC AND RELAXATION

Relaxing music correlates with physical measures associated with relaxation. Listening to relaxing music can help reduce blood pressure, improve immune system functioning, and have other positive effects to help reduce the strains of disease or prevent disease (Pothoulaki, MacDonald, and Flowers 2012).

Music associated with relaxation is characterized by more variation, fluctuations in the loudness pattern, an upbeat tone, a longer melodic tempo, and a transparent and bright tone. Hard rock, rap, and techno-sounds (pop-tech) are created to arouse and activate, and this class of music is least relaxing (Leman et al. 2013). However, abrupt changes from fast music to slow, sad music can promote relaxed feelings (van der Zwaag et al. 2013).

Music that is self-selected for its calming effect can produce physiological changes that are consistent with calm feelings (van der Zwaag et al. 2012). Self-selected classical music may have a calming effect (Trappe 2009).

Music is also available in nature, of course, including birdsong and myriad other sounds that you can hear only when you get outdoors and into a quiet enough place to listen. Although the right music can tone down your psychobiological stress system, the natural sound of a rippling brook can be even more effective (Thoma et al. 2013).

EXERCISE: COMBINING SCENIC VIEWS AND MUSICAL EFFECTS

Pick five scenes that you like and five musical pieces that you like. Test all combinations. Rank them. Pick best combinations. Use one top combination for five minutes twice a day (morning and late afternoon). The next day, repeat this sequence with another top combination.

Continue to do this daily for as long as you like. Experiment to see what you find most relaxing.

With a relaxed body, you are likely to have thoughts that fit the mood. This experience has a restorative value. When relaxed, you are less likely to worry, and that is a good thing.

YOUR PROGRESS REPORT

Write down what you learned from this chapter and what actions you plan to take. Then record what resulted from taking these actions and what you've gained.

What are three key ideas that you took away from this chapter?

1.

2.

3.

What top three actions can you take to combat a specific anxiety or fear?

1.

2.

3.

What resulted when you took these actions?

1.

2.

3.

What did you gain from taking action? What would you do differently next time?

1.

2.

3.

CHAPTER 9

Relax Your Body, Relax Your Mind

Although CBT is normally more effective for anxiety than relaxation methods (Cuijpers et al. 2014), relaxation training helps improve your mental flexibility (Lee and Orsillo 2014) and may serve as an effective part of your CBT program. By themselves, relaxation methods have mild to strong effects on reducing anxious tensions (Manzoni et al. 2008) and seem effective for reducing generalized anxiety (Siev and Chambless 2007). When it comes to developing assertiveness skills and controlling phobias, relaxation can be useful in conjunction with exposure methods. This chapter introduces several relaxation methods, including diaphragmatic breathing, visualization, meditation, and mindfulness practices.

BREATHING AND RELAXING

Breathing exercises are simple to learn and can have relatively quick effects. Psychologist Jon Carlson describes a belly-breathing technique that can send calming signals to the brain (see "Foreword"). This technique involves breathing in a way that your belly expands as you breathe in and contracts as you breathe out. According to Carlson, this belly-breathing method produces calm. Slow, diaphragmatic breathing exercises can help promote a feeling of relaxation and improved attention and awareness (Hazlett-Stevens and Craske 2008).

EXERCISE: PRACTICE DIAPHRAGMATIC BREATHING

Follow these steps to practice breathing slowly from your diaphragm:

1. Breathe in so that your belly expands. Hold your hands on your stomach. You should notice your hands moving out.

2. Within about four seconds, take in a full breath.

3. Hold your breath for about four seconds.

4. Exhale over a four-second period.

5. Wait two seconds and then repeat the sequence.

Follow this breathing sequence for two to four minutes, or longer. Some recommend exhaling over eight seconds. Experiment with each step to see what timing and techniques work best for you.

IMAGINATION AND RELAXATION

Using your imagination is a good way to help you relax. One way to relax is to use visualization exercises in which you imagine pleasant, relaxing imagery.

EXERCISE: VISUALIZING PLEASANT SCENES

Find a peaceful place and make yourself comfortable. For about a minute apiece, imagine any or all of the scenes that these questions suggest:

- Can you imagine a yellow kite floating high in the bright blue sky?

- Can you see a yellow rose move gently in a light breeze?

- Can you picture the sight and sounds of a narrow woodland brook running under the boughs of dark green trees?

- Can you see yourself reclining restfully in a rocking chair in a quiet room?

- Can you imagine an aquarium with brightly colored tropical fish swimming about?

- Can you imagine your body feeling like a limp rag doll?

- Can you imagine dusting of mist hovering over a green summer meadow?

- Can you imagine a falling leaf gently rocking downward in the air?

- Can you imagine the word RELAX written in soft green letters?

Can you feel the sensations of inner peace? If certain suggestions especially appeal to you, then spend more time with the related imagery. Don't concern yourself with how well you are doing as you do this exercise. There is no right way to do it. Let the results be your guide.

Another way to use your imagination to relax is the quartz stone technique.

EXERCISE: USING THE QUARTZ STONE TECHNIQUE

Find a small quartz stone that can easily fit inside your hand (actually any small stone will do). Now take these steps.

1. Pretend the stone is like a diode, where current flows in only one direction.

2. Hold your stone tight. Then very slowly loosen your grip on the stone until you are cradling it in your hand. As you slowly ease your grip, imagine your tension flowing into the stone.

3. Imagine that as the stone draws the tension from your body, it stays trapped in the stone.

4. After about two minutes, toss the stone with its stored tension.

As an alternative to imagining tension flowing from your body to the stone, you can imagine the stone gradually drawing the flow of your anxious thoughts to itself.

MEDITATION

Among the different relaxation techniques, meditation methods generally pull the strongest relaxation effects (Manzoni et al. 2008). Meditation is a traditional Buddhist way of feeling in harmony with yourself and the world around you. Straightforward meditation methods are generally more effective than the more complex, ritualistic variety (Eppley, Abrams, and Shear 1989).

Psychologically stressed persons who participated in an extensive eight-week mindfulness-based stress reduction (MBSR) program based on Jon Kabat-Zinn's (1990) work showed improved memory, learning, emotional regulation, and perspective; also increased brain gray matter associated with brain regions responsible for these functions (Hölzel et al. 2011). Loving-kindness meditation (LKM) also showed increases in gray matter in brain areas related to empathy and emotional regulation (Leung et al. 2013). People use LKM to deepen a sense of unconditional kindness to all people.

Mindfulness-based therapy may be as effective as cognitive behavioral therapy in reducing anxiety, depression, and stress (Khoury et al. 2013). However, mindfulness meditation methods might be inflated by other conditions (Eberth and Sedlmeier 2012). For example, a nonjudgmental approach may contribute to a tranquility effect.

EXERCISE: A BASIC MEDITATION METHOD

Plan on taking ten minutes to test this simple meditation method. You can be sitting, lying down, leaning against a wall, or walking down a wooded path. Operate in what you find to be a comfortable posture and peaceful place.

1. When you are comfortable, repeat a single-syllable word or sound such as "ohm." This is your mantra, or chant. Stretch out the word. For example, ohm stretches out to "ohmmmmm."

2. Breathe in slowly and then slowly exhale. As you breathe in, think "ohhhhh" in a sort of humming tone. As you exhale, extend this to "mmmmmmm." Continue this sequence every ten to fifteen seconds for this ten-minute period.

3. If your mind drifts, go back to repeating your word.

It can be challenging to concentrate on one word without your mind drifting to other thoughts. Don't try to force other thoughts out of your awareness. Your only task during this time is to repeat the word.

If you choose to practice meditating, plan to do this exercise twice a day for the next eight weeks. Pick a time that works for you, such as early morning and late afternoon. See what happens.

Top Tip: Fear Is Not a Permanent Fixture

Atlanta psychotherapist Ed Garcia suggests that the harder you try to avoid fear, the more fear can dominate your life. Garcia suggests that you consider this question: Rather than view fear as something to get rid of, what if you welcomed fear and invited it along in your journey through life? Think of your fear thought(s) as a passenger on this journey, not a permanent fixture in it.

MINDFULNESS-BASED COGNITIVE THERAPY

Mindfulness-based cognitive therapy (MBCT) combines nonjudgmental Buddhist and cognitive therapy methods. You view your unwanted thoughts as messages that pass through your mind: you're not stuck with them. MBCT shows promise for reducing tension (Bishop 2007), general anxiety (Evans et al. 2008), mixed anxiety and depression (Galante, Iribarren, and Pearce 2013), and anxiety and depression about cancer treatment and relapse (Piet, Würtzen, and Zachariae

2012). You can engage a mindfulness view whenever unwanted thoughts are going through your mind. Here are five acceptances that support this process:

1. Accept that anxious exaggerations are mental events that do not define your global self.

2. Accept that anxious thoughts and feelings are transitory events. Like storms, they pass.

3. Accept that anxious thoughts that exist in the present moment do not guarantee what will happen next.

4. Accept that life includes unpleasant events and sufferings that come and go like passing winds.

5. Gestalt therapy founder Fritz Perls (1973) taught that instead of defining certain thoughts or feelings as alien parts of your being, you accept them rather than disown them. Your thoughts and feelings come from you. They are part of you for the moment. But they are not the whole of you.

Top Tip: Use Cognitive Defusion to Avoid Buying Into Negative Thoughts

Dr. Steven C. Hayes, Foundation Professor of Psychology, University of Nevada, codeveloper of acceptance and commitment therapy, and the author of *Get Out of Your Mind and Into Your Life*, shares his top tip for defusing negative thinking.

"In our normal mode of mind, thoughts are what they say they are. If you think you are bad, then you are. If you think life is not worth living, it isn't. If you think anxiety is horrible, it is. Defusion methods are not designed to eliminate thoughts but to help people see thoughts as thoughts, so a greater sense of choice is possible. Instead of being dictated to by the mind, or running on mental 'automatic pilot,' defusion methods help us back up a step or two and be able to see mental operations in flight, and not necessarily act on them, argue with them, resist them, or do what they say. Instead, we can notice them, learn what we can from them, and then direct our attention toward what brings meaning, vitality, and purpose into our lives.

"To see how defusion methods work, think of one of your classic, habitual, judgmental negative thoughts about yourself or your life. Pick one of the old ones: things like *I will never be good enough*, or *I'm different*, or *There is something wrong with me*. Try these things one at a time:

1. Imagine yourself at a very young age. Picture that child in front of you, and when you have that image clear, have the child say the difficult thought out loud. How would

you show compassion for a child of that age who thought such a painful thing? How can you show the same compassion for yourself now when you have such a thought?

2. Form the difficult thought clearly in your mind and then sing the thought to the tune of 'Happy Birthday.' As the tune carries the thought along, consider whether this old automatic thought is really your enemy or whether you can let it sit there like you might an old song.

3. Think the thought again, but add these words at the beginning: 'I'm having the thought that…' If you notice reactions that follow (additional thoughts or emotions), label them too (for example, 'I'm having the feeling of sadness').

4. Distill the thought down to one or two words (for example, if the thought is *I'm a loser*, distill it down to "loser"). Now say that thought as fast as you can out loud for thirty seconds. As the word begins to lose meaning, and you begin to notice how it sounds and what it feels like to say it, gently consider whether it works to let what is, at its base, a sound and a movement run your life.

"Once you see how the mind pulls off the illusion of literal meaning, you can make up your own methods to put your own mental machinery on a leash. These methods work best if they are used as ways of helping you to see how the mind uses sleight-of-hand tricks to pull off its central illusion. If they are used as a means to eliminate, ridicule, or subtract your difficult thoughts, they tend not to work as well, and the reason is this: it means you are buying into another thought (the one that says that this other thought needs to go away!). Defusion is not about winning a mental war; it's about stepping off that field of battle."

YOUR PROGRESS REPORT

Write down what you learned from this chapter and what actions you plan to take. Then record what resulted from taking these actions and what you've gained.

What are three key ideas that you took away from this chapter?

1.

2.

3.

What top three actions can you take to combat a specific anxiety or fear?

1.

2.

3.

What resulted when you took these actions?

1.

2.

3.

What did you gain from taking action? What would you do differently next time?

1.

2.

3.

CHAPTER 10

How to Break a Cognition-Anxiety Connection

Las Vegas psychologist Jon Geis (personal communication) tells a story of identical twins on an ocean beach. One jumps up and down with glee. He speeds toward the waves yelling "Whoopee!" The other clings to his mother. She holds his hand and tries to bring him to the water. His eyes well up with tears, and he digs his heels into the sand.

Why the difference in how the twins react to the water? One boy sees the water as fun whereas the other sees it as a threat. How we perceive things affects how we feel. Geis is not alone in making this point:

- The Greek philosopher Aristotle said that people think themselves into superiority, anger, and shame (Jebb 1909).

- The ancient Stoics viewed emotional distress as triggered by false judgments (Epictetus 2004).

- Psychologist Magna Arnold (1960) proposed that emotion arises from appraisals of events.

- Psychologist Richard Lazarus (Lazarus and Lazarus 1994) viewed emotions as triggered by appraisals where we take our well-being into account.

Emotions from our prehistoric past remain while other emotions reflect our modern social learnings, beliefs, and appraisals. When it comes to coping with anxieties and fears, it's important to take both our primitive emotions and our modern appraisal-based emotions into account.

A FIVE-STEP METACOGNITIVE APPROACH

Your actions and emotions are appropriate to whatever you are thinking. But is your thinking appropriate? Feelings of distress that arise from faulty interpretations and beliefs warrant review.

When your anxieties reflect how you define, appraise, and judge an anxiety-activating situation, do a metacognitive reappraisal. Follow a reflective sequence where you think about your thinking, ferret out beliefs that stir anxiety, and instruct yourself on how to eliminate your false beliefs. A surprising number of people skip this sequence of steps.

How can you tell when you are thinking anxious thoughts? You can tell by their results. You feel them! Use the following five-step metacognitive approach to recognize and then defuse anxiety thinking.

1. Identify your *anxiety activator*—whatever stimulates anxious feelings, such as a change in your mood or anticipation of a situation that you dread.

2. Reflect on what you are perceiving or believing. Do you exaggerate a danger like the frightened twin at the ocean?

3. Separate fiction from fact. You may see an upcoming situation as something that can overwhelm you. Write down what you have to be telling yourself to feel overwhelmed. Are you telling yourself that *This is too much for me?* If so, what is too much? Is it the tension?

4. Reappraise your situation from a coping perspective. This is where you look at reasonable and realistic alternative possibilities that counteract parasitic anxiety beliefs.

5. Act to develop emotional tolerance by allowing yourself to experience emotions, such as anxiety, fear, and depression, that you think you can't stand feeling.

Top Tip: Be Mindful of What You Are Doing

San Diego, California Archpriest Dr. George Morelli is a clinical psychologist and the author of *Healing—Volume 2: Reflections for Clergy, Chaplains, and Counselors.* George shares a mindfulness tip:

"The behavioral research literature supports a clinical tool called *mindfulness* which can be used to break bad habits and overcome troublesome emotions, such as anxiety. Mindfulness is 'the awareness that emerges through paying attention on purpose, in the present moment, and nonjudgmentally to the unfolding of experience moment by moment' (Kabat-Zinn 2003, 145).

"To follow a mindfulness way,

1. Focus on the sensory and physical aspects of the present moment.

2. Recognize thought patterns, feelings, and physical sensations that are occurring, and learn to tell the difference between sensation, thoughts, and feelings.

3. Practice making decisions based on the choices you want, that feel right, and that won't needlessly interfere with the rights of others.

"By keeping your eyes on the target—what you want to accomplish—anxieties and fears become transparent barriers that you can move through on your way to pursuing a greater cause or purpose."

• *Ken's Story*

A client named Ken suffered from anxiety after his long-term girlfriend broke up with him. Ken felt devastated and depressed by the loss. He felt anxious that he would never find anyone to love. He used a five-step metacognitive approach to defuse his anxiety over the loss and to free himself from needless anguish.

Ken's Five Metacognitive Steps to Boost Emotional Tolerance for Anxiety over Loss

1. **Identify anxiety activator.**	The love of Ken's life broke up with him and went off to date someone else.
2. **Reflect on cognitive triggers and amplifiers.**	Ken wrote out his thoughts, and this exercise helped him hone in on a dire prediction. He worried that he would never find anyone else. This thought of growing old was more than worrisome. It became his reality.
3. **Separate fiction from fact.**	Ken separated the parts of his thinking that were factual from the parts that he exaggerated. Fact: He felt upset about the betrayal and that he didn't see it coming. Losses of this sort are rarely welcome. However, thinking that he would never find another person to love and would grow old alone was dramatic and unprovable.

4. **Reappraise your situation from a coping perspective.**	Ken first reappraised his status by looking at alternative possibilities: (1) Is it possible to accept the sadness of the loss and to live beyond it? (2) Is it possible to think clearly about a loss and betrayal and still feel emotionally saddened? (3) Is it possible to eventually get beyond the feeling of loss and to find someone to both trust and love?
5. **Develop tolerance tactics.**	(1) Ken picked an hour each day for five days in a row when he allowed himself to feel the loss. He was less likely to dramatize the loss when he chose to disentangle himself from the complications of the betrayal and accept his sadness. (2) He came to accept that his sadness arose from his memories. He had a lot of different memories that fed into his sense of loss and sadness. (3) With each memory, he implanted a realistic, moderate affective label to describe the experience, such as "I enjoyed that experience and can still enjoy the memory despite the loss." This form of affective labeling doesn't soft-pedal the betrayal or diminish the sadness of loss. Rather, it's an acceptance that both experiences are part of the same memory picture.

Betrayals and losses are complex. Anger, anxieties, self-doubts, and recriminations were part of Ken's bundle of emotions. But time does heal most wounds. Situational emotions that were once live issues eventually fade. Torments become tolerable. Lessons learned carry over to the next situation. Life goes on.

EXERCISE: YOUR FIVE-STEP METACOGNITIVE APPROACH

Now it's your turn to try the five-step metacognitive approach. Pick a problem. Tune into your anxious thinking. Confront anxiety from a metacognitive perspective, separating facts from fictions (watch for exaggerations). Act to develop a coping perspective by decreasing needless negatives and by recognizing different parts of a bigger picture. Act to develop an inner tolerance without attempting to suppress emotions that are appropriate to the situation. Use the chart provided to record your progress.

Five Metacognitive Steps to Boost Emotional Tolerance

1. Identify anxiety activator.	
2. Reflect on cognitive triggers and amplifiers.	
3. Separate fiction from fact.	
4. Reappraise your situation from a coping perspective.	
5. Develop tolerance tactics.	

Emotions may be natural, they may trigger thoughts about themselves, or they may emerge based on how you appraise a situation. Cognitive appraisals and emotions may also feed off each other. Let's turn to that matter next.

BREAKING CIRCULAR-THINKING PATTERNS

Anxiety commonly follows a circular-thinking cycle. You engage in circular thinking when your emotions validate an erroneous premise: *I fear the presence of a ghost under my bed. Because I feel this feeling, there is a ghost under my bed.* Well, that circularity is a tad extreme. Using a feeling to validate a belief that evokes it is a dubious practice.

Here is a common circular loop: You face a personally relevant but uncertain situation. You anticipate an awful result. You feel anxious. You act as if your feelings of anxiety validate the worst-case scenario.

One way to break out of the circle is to pause long enough to notice that your thinking is circular. If you preface your conclusion with the phrase "I assume" (*Because I feel fear, I assume there is a ghost under my bed*), you may be able to prevent the idea from becoming an uncontested conviction.

USING YOUR IMAGINATION TO CONTROL ANXIETY

When you feel anxious about the same things, tune in to yourself. The odds are that you'll hear anxiety scripts that are built around cognitive and behavioral themes. If so, you can then rewrite your own script to bring about a functional new narrative.

EXERCISE: ASSERT YOURSELF

Imagine yourself surrounded by your anxieties, with each one playing a part in a daily performance. Among the actors, you have social anxiety, anxiety over uncertainty, fear of loss of control, and many other discordant characters, each with a special script to read. Give each one a name. Imagine each form of anxiety reading from a script in an ongoing television series. What is the main theme for each script? Is it exaggeration? What is the beginning, the middle, and the end?

Try giving each voice of anxiety a voice of someone you don't respect. Can a shift in tone make your voice of anxiety sound unappealing?

Now, make your voice of reason into a main character. Write reason into the script. What does this character called Reason think? What does Reason feel? What does Reason do? Here's a suggestion: When you rewrite the script, act as if you were the master of your fate, and then quell any debate with your anxiety characters by describing why this is so. For example, you can change your thinking, you can tolerate tension, and you can act in your best interest.

Here's another idea: You might ask each anxiety, "Why would you act to prevent positive change and progress?" Answers based on flimsy logic are open to special scrutiny. Rebut them.

By confronting your anxieties in this way, you can gain a different perspective. You can also use your imagination to give the voice of reason a bigger role. If you evoke the image of reason when you experience anxiety and fear thinking, you may find it easier to change your anxiety script.

RESOLVING YOUR APPROACH-AND-AVOIDANCE CONFLICTS

Happiness and anxiety are polar opposites (Lench, Flores, and Bench 2011). Happiness is an approach emotion. Anxiety is an avoidance emotion. Not surprisingly, it's easier to be successful when happy, and happy when successful (Lyubomirsky, King, and Diener 2005). That's because you are inclined to approach opportunities that you associate with thriving and happiness. You would be likely to avoid these same situations if you viewed them as threats.

When you fear what you want, you may feel caught between a rock and a hard place. For example, you want something, but you associate discomfort with approaching what you want, and you want to avoid feeling uncomfortable. Now you have an approach-avoidance conflict. If you can teach yourself to approach worthy challenges that you'd ordinarily avoid, you will increase your chances for success and happiness. There are many ways to do this. One way is to weigh your options.

EXERCISE: SCALE OF JUSTICE

Think of a worthy goal that you have anxieties about pursuing. For example, you have an interview for a job that you want (approach condition). You're afraid you'll mess up the interview (avoidance condition). You are straddled between desire and anxiety. You feel stuck. How do you resolve this classic approach-avoidance conflict?

Pretend that you are holding a scale of justice. On one side of the scale, you have "approach," and on the other side you have "avoidance." Logically, approaching your goal is more important than avoiding the fear, yet fear currently feels heavier. Can you tip the balance in favor of approach?

Imagine that the benefits of reaching your goal and the benefits of ridding yourself of your fear are each written on small stones. The value of avoidance is written on tissue paper. For every piece of tissue paper, you have a corresponding stone.

Imagine that your stones are each inscribed with a benefit. (If your goal were a new job, these inscriptions might be better pay or better hours. Some benefits of overcoming your fear might be better self-control, increased self-efficacy, and less tension from needless fears.) The tissue paper also carries inscriptions, such as relief through avoidance. Write down what's on each side of your scale of justice.

Approach	Avoidance
1.	1.
2.	2.
3.	3.

4.	4.
5.	5.
6.	6.
7.	7.
8.	8.
9.	9.
10.	10.

In this exercise, the benefits of approach outweigh the benefits of avoidance. It's fair to stack the deck in this way, especially if you've stacked it against yourself in the past. Does this image give you a different perspective on how to gain justice for yourself?

Whenever you prioritize avoidance over approaching a goal, keep the scale of justice image in mind. However, you won't get far beyond this intellectual perspective unless you take the necessary steps toward success.

YOUR PROGRESS REPORT

Write down what you learned from this chapter and what actions you plan to take. Then record what resulted from taking these actions and what you've gained.

What are three key ideas that you took away from this chapter?

1.

2.

3.

What top three actions can you take to combat a specific anxiety or fear?

1.

2.

3.

What resulted when you took these actions?

1.

2.

3.

What did you gain from taking action? What would you do differently next time?

1.

2.

3.

CHAPTER 11

Thinking Your Way Out of Anxiety

When you feel anxious, you'll have interconnecting negative thoughts. For example, you may worry about feeling fatigued from losing sleep. That worry may link to anxiety about your fatigue. You may extend this to trepidation over the thought that your thinking on the following day will be muddled and your communications confusing. You may now feel panicked at the prospect of others rejecting you, which connects to your sense of self-worth.

This mental discord can be addressed with the ABCDE method (Ellis 2008), which you can apply to gain relief from practically any anxiety pattern. This chapter offers Fred's anxiety predicament as an example of how the ABCDE method can be used to resolve a complex anxiety problem.

• Fred's Story

Fred was a forty-eight-year-old widower with two grown children. As a successful inventor, he retired with ample financial resources. After his retirement, he spent several hours weekly in volunteer work. He was strongly family oriented. Whenever he had the opportunity, he would spend time with his children and his grandchildren. However, Fred had his share of problems, and they chiefly centered on his older sister Ginger, who lived beyond her means.

Ginger's life revolved around one financial crisis after another. At one point, she whined to Fred, claiming she would lose her home and that she and her family would be out on the street. Fred wrote a check to pay off her second mortgage. Next, her daughter's college tuition was overdue. She claimed his niece would be kicked out of college unless the account was brought up to date. Fred wrote the check. Then her son needed to get a car so that he could deliver pizza. She told Fred that she feared that her son would go back to using cocaine unless he got the job. Fred bought the car.

Fred tried to downplay the extent of his relatives' problems by saying to himself that everyone would eventually come to their senses. This hope was an illusion.

Fred's relationship with his sister and her family was not entirely negative. When his wife was alive, the two families had gone on vacations together. He had good memories of his sister's children growing up and the birthdays and holidays the family had shared together. His children and his sister's children continued to enjoy positive relationships. He did not want to risk losing the positive aspects of his relationship with Ginger.

When Fred and Ginger were children, Ginger was the dominant sibling. Taking advantage of being older, she micromanaged Fred. When Fred was in high school, if Ginger did not like one of his girlfriends, he dropped her.

Ginger did not approve of Fred's new fiancée. This time, Fred decided to take a stand. He refused to leave the woman he loved. Fred hated confrontation of any sort. He entered therapy when his confrontation anxieties felt unbearable.

SETTING GOALS

As you gain perspective on your anxieties, you may realize that you need to make some changes in how you go about your life. Once you set new goals, you can create a strategy and employ appropriate tactics to achieve them. Fred, for example, realized that he was far from taking charge of himself. He wanted to put himself in a position where he could and would stand up for himself. That was his goal. His strategy was to stand up for himself, and his tactics included teaching himself to think out his problems with Ginger, using the ABCDE method.

Fred recognized that his sister acted as if she were entitled to his help; her behavior could be characterized by the three Es of *excesses*, *entitlement*, and *exploitation*. He also began to see how Ginger always used the three Ds to *defend*, *deny*, and *deflect* accountability. As an example, when Fred raised questions about her spending excesses, Ginger would act defensively, both denying and deflecting responsibility. Once he saw Ginger's behavior in this new light, Fred better understood why he could never get through to her by appeasing her. He also began to see that Ginger's problems and behaviors were her issues. How he responded was his issue.

Fred's most pressing concern was his own anxiety. He hated feeling tense over his tension. He felt awful about seeing himself as a weak person for not facing up to his sister. Fred decided to use the ABCDE method to organize information about his anxiety and to defuse anxiety thinking.

USING THE ABCDE METHOD

Albert Ellis's ABCDE method is a common part of most CBT programs and can be used to overcome any parasitic anxiety pattern. The acronym stands for five steps:

A is an *adversity,* or activating event. The first step is to recognize this trigger.

B stands for your *beliefs* about the adversity. These beliefs can range from weakly held ones to strong convictions. They can be reasonable or erroneous or somewhere in between. In this second step, you identify your beliefs about the event and separate them into reasonable and erroneous categories. (Step D gives you criteria for separating reasonable from erroneous beliefs, in a way that can help you develop a realistic perspective about your anxiety situation and gain relief.)

C stands for the emotional and behavioral *consequences* of having beliefs. In this step, you list the consequences of both your reasonable and your erroneous beliefs. For example, a consequence of the belief that you are in threatening emotional circumstances where you are helpless might be one of panic. Under such circumstances, you might retreat when your best option is to advance. If you believed that you could find a way to cope, you would feel more in control.

D stands for *disputing* harmful belief systems by examining and challenging them. In case you are new to this process, this step includes six perspective-generating questions to help you dispute your beliefs. You supply the answers: (1) Does the belief fit with reality (that is, is the belief confirmable through experiment, or is it fact-based)? (2) Does the belief support the achievement of reasonable and constructive interests and goals? (3) Does the belief help foster positive relationships? (4) Does the belief conform to a measurable reality? (5) Does the belief seem reasonable and logical in the context in which it occurs? (6) Is the belief generally helpful or generally detrimental? Once you've mastered this six-step questioning method, you can customize your questions. (See chapters 16 and 22 for further examples of how to dispute anxiety thinking.) This process can lead to a perspective that is relatively free of erroneous beliefs and exaggerations about the evocative situation.

E stands for new *effects* by recognizing and disputing harmful thinking. Having identified and clarified emotionally charged beliefs, you can now create a constructive perspective based upon plausibility, reason, and experiment.

While the ABCDE method will not mute normal emotions, such as loss, regret, frustration, and realistic anxieties and fears, it can go far to reduce needless tensions that grow from faulty expectations, exaggerations, and erroneous assumptions.

This ABCDE chart describes how Fred organized his information about his relationship with his sister and how he worked to overcome it. Fred's most pressing concern was his own anxiety. He hated feeling tense over his tension. He reported feeling awful about seeing himself as a weak person for not facing up to his sister. Thus he focused first on standing up to his sister.

Fred's ABCDE Resolution

Adversity or activating event: *Sister engaging in exploitive manipulations to get "entitlement" dollars to cover financial excesses.*

Reasonable beliefs about the event: I don't like being put into a corner where I capitulate to my sister's insistence and demand for money to bail her out from the consequences of her own excesses.

Emotional and behavioral consequences of the reasoned belief: *Regret, disappointment with sister's behavior, and dislike of the situation.*

Potentially erroneous beliefs about the events: I can't stand up to my sister. *Belief that appeasement will eliminate anxiety.*

Emotional and behavioral consequence of the potentially erroneous beliefs: *Self-loathing for capitulation. Intolerance for tension and retreat from tension.*

Disputing potentially erroneous beliefs: Fred reminded himself of his basic family values. He recognized that he would want to help his sister if she were ill or if she had no control over adverse events, but he did not want to help her repeat what were actually self-destructive habits. With that in mind, Fred asked and answered six questions:

1. "Does my belief that I cannot stand up to my sister fit with reality?"

   Answer: "No. There are exceptions. I married my wife, despite my sister's strong protests, and had a wonderful marriage. I have the power to say no."

2. "Does my belief that I must avoid conflict with my sister over money help me achieve my constructive interests and goals?"

   Answer: "No. It actually defeats my interest in overcoming anxiety related to her demands."

3. "Does my belief in avoiding conflict by capitulation foster a constructive relationship with my sister?"

   Answer: "No. This aspect of my relationship with her is dysfunctional and likely will continue to be as long as she believes she can get whatever she demands from me."

4. "Does my belief that I can't defend myself conform to reality?"

   Answer: "No. The belief that I'm too weak and will be overwhelmed by her if I defend my position is a fear, not a fact."

5. "Does my belief in capitulation seem reasonable and make sense in the context in which it occurs?"

Answer: "No. My sister's excesses, entitlement beliefs, and exploitive manipulations are unreasonable. To avoid conflict, I allow myself to deflate my own sense of self-worth by labeling myself weak and inept. That conclusion is based upon a magical view that my worth depends upon her approval."

6. "Is my appeasement belief generally helpful or detrimental?"

Answer: "In this case, it is generally detrimental. It costs time, emotional energy, and money, with no benefits in return."

Effects of the disputation exercise: A better perspective on the issues. A resolve to refuse Ginger's urgent pressures to bail her out of her financial troubles. A recognition that self-worth does not depend upon capitulation to another's expectations and demands. Self-acceptance with or without sister's approval. Recognition that working on tolerance for tension will help build a sense of inner control.

Using this ABCDE method of analysis gave Fred clarity about his situation. As a result, he took action and stopped capitulating to Ginger's financial demands. He reported feeling relief as a result. He noticed that Ginger started to live within her means. His newfound courage was helpful to her as well.

EXERCISE: ABCDE PRACTICE

Use the ABCDE method to attack your main anxiety. Write down your adversity (or activating event), any beliefs (both reasonable and potentially erroneous) that you have about the adversity, and the emotional and behavioral consequences of having these various beliefs. Then dispute your potentially erroneous beliefs, and see what happens. Finally, write down the effects of this process.

Your ABCDE Resolution

Adversity or activating event:
Reasonable beliefs about the event:
Emotional and behavioral consequences of the reasonable beliefs:
Potentially erroneous beliefs about the event:
Emotional and behavioral consequences of potentially erroneous beliefs:
Disputing potentially erroneous beliefs: 1. Does the belief fit with reality? (Is the belief confirmable through experiment? Is there evidence to support the belief? Is it or is it not fact based?) 2. Does the belief support the achievement of reasonable and constructive interests and goals? 3. Does the belief help foster positive relationships? 4. Does the belief conform to a measurable reality? 5. Does the belief seem reasonable and logical in the context in which it occurs? 6. Is the belief generally detrimental or generally helpful?
Effects of the disputation exercise:

Top Tip: Melt Anxiety with Mindfulness and Rational Thinking

Dr. Vincent E. Parr is a psychologist in private practice in Tampa. Michael Gregory, a former Buddhist monk, directs the Mindfulness Meditation Center in Palmetto, Florida. Together, they offer this top tip for combining rational and mindfulness methods:

"If you suffer from a parasitic form of anxiety, attack it using a combined mindfulness and rational-thinking approach. Start by matching your what-if-thinking against this anxiety equation: A = WI + Aw + ICSI, where

A = Anxiety, or a negative feeling of dread

WI = What-if-thinking that something very bad, dangerous, or threatening could happen to you or to someone you love

Aw = Awfulizing, or emotionally blowing up a real or imagined situation by defining it as awful, terrible, or horrible

ICSI = 'I can't stand it,' where you believe that you can't tolerate the unpleasant feelings.

Accept that you've concocted a future event (WI), scared yourself about this possibility (Aw), and viewed yourself as unable to stand the emotions about an event that you have no proof exists (ICSI).

How can you stop tormenting yourself with what-if-thinking?

- Recognize that parasitic anxiety takes place in your mind, and allow yourself—without struggle—to observe WI anxiety as it unfolds.

- Remind yourself to remain mindful, which is a nonreactive and nonjudgmental awareness of self and surroundings.

- Accept that WI parasitic thinking is a mental projection that connects horrifying thoughts and images to anxiety, but thinking about a WI disaster doesn't validate the disaster.

- Release the image of your expected disaster by allowing it to pass through your mind as an errant neuron discharge.

- Shift from a passive to an active perspective. Talk to yourself in a realistic and self-assuring way. For example, 'Parasitic anxiety is fertilized by thoughts and images. This anxiety doesn't exist without the passing thoughts or images that accompany anxiety.'

- Use a coping statement to challenge both Aw and ICSI thinking. For example, 'Even if what I imagined did happen, it would only be as awful as I think. I can stand—albeit unhappily—what I don't like.' (Appropriate coping statements are research-supported ways to down-regulate negative affect, such as anxiety.)"

YOUR PROGRESS REPORT

Write down what you learned from this chapter and what actions you plan to take. Then record what resulted from taking these actions and what you've gained.

What are three key ideas that you took away from this chapter?

1.

2.

3.

What top three actions can you take to combat a specific anxiety or fear?

1.

2.

3.

What resulted when you took these actions?

1.

2.

3.

What did you gain from taking action? What would you do differently next time?

1.

2.

3.

CHAPTER 12

Behavioral Methods to Defeat Fear

Exposure is a critical part of a cognitive, emotive, and behavioral approach to overcoming fears, phobias, and panic. This is a form of learning where you repeatedly put yourself in proximity to a feared situation. Through this habituation process, you retrain your brain to stop being so overreactive to nondangerous situations.

This chapter looks at the exposure programs of Judy, Dell, and Sandra, all of whom had crippling fears that they were able to overcome. You can use aspects of these programs that you believe will work for you.

OVERCOMING PHOBIAS

Phobias, like fear of heights or fear of the dark, can start at any point in life, but often they start in childhood, when we cannot discern rational from irrational beliefs and fears. If these fears continue into adulthood, then you may realize that your fear is irrational but maintain the fear by continuing to avoid any situation that triggers it.

• Judy's Story

Ever since she was a child, Judy had a morbid fear of darkness. She thought it started from a story her uncle told her about "the bogeys." These were apparitions who flew invisibly through the darkness to steal the souls of little children who misbehaved. After hearing that story, she recalled feeling petrified of the dark. She knew she wasn't perfect, and she figured the bogeys would come to get her.

To help quell her fears, her father suggested that she keep a light on in her room. Her mother said, "The bogeys can't get you in the light." This calmed her. But she continued to have a morbid fear of being in the dark and of having her soul torn away by invisible bogeys.

Judy worried about what would happen if the lights went out and she had no safe place to hide. She solved this problem by having backup systems. She kept candles and a battery-operated lantern in her bedroom. Her parents thought this was excessive. They also believed she would grow out of her fears, but Judy's fear of darkness continued into adulthood.

Of course, the bogey story was silly. Judy figured this out around the same time she stopped believing in the tooth fairy. Yet her fear of the dark continued. Her fear affected her social life. As a young teen, Judy refused to go to summer camp, because she knew that there would come a time when the lights would go out. She wanted to avoid panicking and being ridiculed by her peers. For the same reason, she refused to go to sleepovers with her friends. As a young adult, she missed going to her best friend's wedding reception because it was held at night. She wanted to avoid panicking and being ridiculed by her peers.

Her fear generalized to other conditions of darkness, such as driving at night or through dimly lit tunnels. She believed she'd be safe with the dome light on in her car. When asked out on dates, she automatically refused. She feared that she'd expose her fear of darkness to her date. Judy likened her fear of darkness to an alien force that overcame her at night. As a twenty-six-year-old, Judy continued to sleep with a lamp on.

To the outside world, Judy looked as though she lived a normal life. If you didn't know about her fear of the dark, you'd think she was a lovely, upbeat young woman without a care in the world. She had attended day college and received a degree in journalism. She did freelance editing for a major publication house. Meanwhile, Judy continued to live with her parents, who encouraged her to get help for dealing with her dread of darkness. She decided to see if she could find a way to break free from her fear.

A Time-and-Proximity Plan for Defeating Fear

Oftentimes, fears may be so deeply engrained that defeating them requires addressing them on many levels.

In Judy's case, a combined cognitive, emotional tolerance, and behavioral exposure approach held promise. To combat her fear of darkness, she outlined a plan that included both time and proximity dimensions. This plan included addressing her strong tendency to create double troubles by declaring herself a weak person and blaming herself for her problems.

Judy's Time-and-Proximity Plan

Fear of Darkness Dimensions	Cognitive	Emotional Tolerance	Behavioral
Time Dimension	Counteract double troubles and anxiety-and-fear thinking.	Refuse to accept thinking that you can't stand tension.	Design an exposure plan to progressively master a fear of darkness through taking graduated steps to bring about that result.
Proximity Dimension	Tackle fear thoughts that can trigger a feeling of fear and evoke impulses to escape.	Use your intelligence, ingenuity, and will to live through tension for purposes of defeating fear.	Directly face fear by progressively experiencing fear of the dark but under conditions where you are in charge of what you do.

Employing Cognitive and Emotional Tolerance Tactics

Before confronting your fear through exposure, you may need to address certain cognitive or emotional issues that are in the way. For example, after Judy recognized that she was double-troubling herself, she decided to contest this thinking. First, she adopted the slogan "tolerance tames fear," giving herself the right to have a fear habit and a means of dealing with it. Operating from that perspective, she used some cognitive interventions to defuse her double troubles:

- Judy had been seeing herself as a weak person for having a fear of darkness, but downing herself in this way was creating a double trouble. In Judy's mind, her fear of darkness was a sign of weakness, a character flaw. In time, however, she came to accept—not just parrot—that having a foolish fear was a bad-thinking habit. She realized that she had called herself weak to explain why she'd felt afraid. By redefining her fear of darkness as a learned habit, she felt that she could learn to break the habit.

- Judy feared going crazy. Judy thought that her fear could cause her to lose her sense of self and that she would lose her mind. When she learned that a fear of going crazy was a common phobia and even had a name—phrenophobia—this fear quickly vanished. Instead, she came to view her fear of darkness as highly unpleasant. This description better fit with reality.

- Judy had been blaming herself for losing opportunities because of her fear. Blame, in this instance, added surplus meaning to an already unfortunate situation. Damning herself about lost opportunities was like living life in reverse gear. The past wasn't going to change. Judy realized that although the past was gone, she could reexamine and reinterpret events. Although she couldn't go back to do things differently, she could start today to live her life differently.

Working to diminish her double troubles, Judy learned that she felt more tolerant of herself and less worried about feeling fearful. It was time to apply her new beliefs to the challenge of addressing her fear of darkness.

Using a Graduated Exposure Technique

Again, the key to overcoming an irrational fear is to experience the fear; by gradually putting yourself in the situation that you fear, you can see that there is nothing to fear.

Judy's solution for overcoming her fear of darkness therefore involved being in the dark. She expected to show herself that neither darkness nor panic about being in the dark would do her in. She was prepared to deal with the proximity issue where the darker it got, the greater her fear.

A big part of an ongoing fear involves a sense of being out of control and powerless. But what happens when you have a way to assert control? Will that change your perception of the situation? Judy already knew the answer to this question. Though terrified of the dark, Judy had always enjoyed reading horror stories about things that go bump in the night. When reading scary stories, she always knew she could choose to close the book; and because she knew she had this control, she didn't need to exercise it. Judy found that she liked this idea, that she could control aspects of darkness. Judy decided to try a graduated exposure to darkness, in which she would learn to tolerate feelings of tension in manageable doses. The plan enabled her to gradually increase her own exposure to her feared situation.

Judy began using a dimmer switch at night in her bedroom to regulate the level of illumination. She started with the light fully bright. By design, she gradually dialed down the intensity of the light. When she felt tense, she did not increase the level of the light but stayed with the feeling of tension until it lifted. She discovered then that her tension didn't last. She found this phase of exposure easier than she had expected.

With the dimmer switch in hand, Judy felt in control. But at one point she lost this feeling and turned on the light. Setbacks like this are not unusual in exposure programs and can easily be addressed. Judy simply returned to her bedroom an hour later and restarted exposure. This time she kept the light on a bit brighter until she felt comfortable at that level. Then she turned the switch down another notch. She found that she no longer felt a need to escape.

After ten days of progressively dimming the light, Judy could turn out the light and stay in darkness for a minute before she started to feel tense. She increased the amount of time she stayed in darkness in three-minute increments. When Judy achieved the milestone of remaining six minutes in darkness, she began using a dim night-light in her bedroom instead of the higher intensity lamp that she was accustomed to using. After three weeks, Judy shut off the night-light and fell asleep in darkness. Thereafter, she could have the night-light on or keep it off.

Through exposure, Judy showed herself that her fear sensations were time limited and tolerable. She learned she could stand experiencing fear sensations. She felt a huge sense of accomplishment.

Addressing Related Fears

One criticism of behavioral exposure methods is that what you learn in one situation normally won't transfer automatically to another. Judy found that after learning to sleep with the light off, she could go into a dark basement without too much trepidation. She had worked things out in her mind where she knew she could tolerate her fear sensations. However, she was still afraid of driving at night, so she decided to address this fear next. But now she knew what to do and what to expect.

To address her fear of driving at night, she attached opaque plastic sheets to the dome light in her car, so that she could gradually lower the light level until she could drive at night without the dome light on. She repeated the process when driving through tunnels. Within a week, she was driving at night without the dome light and she could drive through tunnels.

A Cognitive, Emotive, Behavioral Plan

This list of actions summarizes the cognitive, emotive, behavioral plan that Judy applied to overcome her fear of darkness:

- Attack double troubles whenever this form of thinking arises.

- Design an exposure sequence that is broken into manageable phases.

- Start with the least intense phase and stick with it until mastered. Then move on to the next.

- Pace yourself. There is no hurry. It takes time for the brain to integrate new information from experience.

- If you have a setback, try again, perhaps with a modified plan.

You can follow these basic steps as you outline your own exposure programs.

What can you do with your time and your life after you are no longer limited because of your fears? In Judy's case, she dated. She attended night courses in journalism. She obtained a master's degree. She went on vacations, something she had not done before. She had her share of setbacks and losses. Nevertheless, she experienced her life as exciting and meaningful.

Top Tip: Expose Yourself Despite the Fear

Distinguished Professor of Psychology at the University of Scranton, psychologist, and author Dr. John Norcross shares this tip on how to take advantage of exposure therapy:

"Every anxious bone in your body is pleading with you to avoid the anxiety: *Run away! Don't even think about it!* Our brains are hardwired to maximize pleasure and to avoid pain.

"But avoidance builds and builds, becoming its own problem and worsening the anxiety. Avoidance is the hallmark of self-defeating behavior.

"The healthy opposite of avoidance is exposure: directly confronting the dreaded situation. It's not as simple as 'Just do it' or as melodramatic as 'Throw them into the deep end of the pool,' but a series of learnable skills: learning to relax; gradual exposure to the fear; not prematurely escaping from the fearful situation.

"And, as you have undoubtedly learned from your childhood experiences, the once-gigantic fear becomes quite manageable within minutes or a couple of hours. Avoidance, by contrast, lasts a lifetime.

"Expose yourself slowly and by leveraging decades of research in doing it most effectively. Remember to relax before confronting the fearful situation. The first few exposures might proceed better if you have a trusted friend or mentor along. If your anxiety remains intense, then expose yourself initially in your imagination until you become less fearful, and then approach the situation. Don't escape from the situation too quickly—it will only intensify the fear in the long run. Remain until you achieve a 50 percent reduction in the anxiety. That way, you will experience the progress and begin transforming those catastrophic worries into realistic can-do thoughts. Finally, bring out the huge rewards for facing the fear and practicing exposure anyway! You deserve it for succeeding despite our hardwired avoidance."

THE BEHAVIORAL CARD-SORT TECHNIQUE

The behavioral card-sort technique can be especially helpful for those who suffer from agoraphobia, who want to overcome panic and fear about being in proximity to "unsafe" locations. The approach is simple:

1. You identify a primary location that triggers fear.

2. You imagine a range of proximities to that location, from the safest to the most dreaded proximity.

3. You write these locations on an index card.

4. You write different proximity conditions on index cards.

5. You sort the cards to develop a list of ranked items from least to most fearsome.

You now have a map set out in graduated steps—from least to most fearsome—that you can follow to progressively master your fear of being in "unsafe" locations.

• Del's Story

Del was a thirty-five-year-old undergraduate biology major. He panicked if he went into a classroom where he did not have the seat closest to the classroom door. He wanted to be close to the door so that he could quickly exit the building should he suffer a panic reaction during the class. His primary fear was that of not being able to escape if he panicked. The farther he was from the exit, the greater his fear.

To avoid panicking over not getting "his seat," Del habitually arrived twenty minutes early for class. Proximity to the door was critical to him. That was his safety blanket.

Being close to an exit was only the tip of the iceberg, however. His fears increased on higher floors. Thus he selected a local college based on the height of the buildings. The science building, where his major subjects were taught, had three stories. When the classes he needed to take were scheduled on the first floor, he'd take them. Otherwise, he'd wait.

With a small family inheritance, Del originally had no need to work. But his inheritance would eventually run out. That reality, along with being fed up with his fears, prompted a decision to act to stop feeling afraid.

Using the Card-Sort Technique

The card-sort technique is helpful for organizing how you will proceed through exposure, especially when there are multiple variables. Del's card-sort technique provides a good example of how it can work. His card-sort ranking involved three classroom locations and five proximity conditions. The locations were the first, second, and third floors of the science building. Del defined his proximity conditions based on distance from the door in each classroom. His least intense proximity condition was attending a class on the first floor and sitting two seats away from the door in the row closest to the door. His most intense proximity condition was sitting in the center of the middle row in a third-floor classroom.

Del devised a graduated exposure plan with location and proximity conditions that went from least to most severe.

Location Conditions

1. First floor

2. Second floor

3. Third floor

Proximity Conditions

1. Two seats away from door in row closest to door

2. Two rows from the door in seat closest to the door

3. Five rows from door in seat closest to door

4. Five rows from the door, middle seat

5. Center of middle row (farthest from the door)

Del started his behavioral card-sort exposure sessions in the spring semester. That spring, he took four courses on the first floor of the same building. This provided ample learning opportunities; he could repeat the card-sort plan daily. He started with the first location and proximity condition and mastered it at his own pace. When he felt reasonably comfortable with step 1, he took the second proximity step, which was to sit two rows from the door in the seat closest to the door. By the end of the semester, Del could comfortably sit anywhere in the first-floor classroom. He was pleased with the results of his exposure program.

For the summer semester, Del enrolled in courses taught on the second and third floors. He decided to use the break between semesters to address his fears of being in the classrooms on these higher floors. The first challenge was to get up the stairs to the second and third floors. For this purpose, Del hired a psychology graduate student as a helper. The student first walked with him up the stairs, providing a sense of security. Next, the student followed thirty seconds behind Del, then one minute behind him, then two minutes, and then not at all. Del repeated this *time-lag technique* going from the second to the third floors. Within a week, he found that he could walk on his own up to the third floor.

As an experiment, Del entered the second- and third-floor classrooms when they were empty. Starting with the second-floor room, he switched seats according to the card-sort plan. Then he sat in every seat in the room (about thirty) for about a minute each. He repeated this exercise on the third floor. He reported feeling bored with the redundancy, but he also reported an absence of fear.

When he began his classes, he did so with some trepidation. The presence of a professor and students in the classroom had a greater impact than he'd expected. It was in these circumstances that he most feared having a panic attack.

To face his fear of panic, Del thought through his fears of what others might think if they saw him panicking. He faced an incongruity: if different people can view the same situation in different ways, why would the members of his class see him only as he saw himself? He accepted that many of his classmates would likely not notice him even if he did feel panicky and that, if the worst happened (if he panicked in the class and was unable to exit), he could still unconditionally accept his fallible self. That insight gave him a positive new perspective.

A week after classes started, Del reported that he could comfortably sit anywhere in either class. He had gotten past a significant hurdle toward finishing his degree.

Coping with Other Factors

Sometimes you may have to deal with other fear factors besides location and proximity conditions. For example, Del was also afraid of being in restaurants where he could not control his seating position, and the bigger the crowd was, the greater his degree of distress. That is, people conditions (fewer or more people present) were a factor in his fear of being in restaurants. Now he had a three-factor problem to resolve.

For his second graded exposure experiment, Del chose a fast-food restaurant. He used the following card-sort ranking system:

Location Conditions	People Conditions	Proximity Conditions
Fast-food restaurant	1. Almost empty	1. Seat close to door
	2. Moderately crowded	2. Seat in middle of restaurant
	3. Crowded	3. Seat farthest from the door

His least worrisome condition was sitting close to the door when the restaurant was nearly empty. The most worrisome condition was sitting in the farthest seat from the door when the restaurant was crowded. Interestingly, Del expressed no fear of going to the counter to order food. The counter was far from the door, but he believed that being on his feet made a difference.

Otherwise, he had no explanation. However, the fact of his ease at the counter caused him to rethink his assumption that he needed to be close to the door.

Within three weeks of this graduated exposure experiment, Del stopped worrying about where he sat in the restaurant.

Using the card-sort technique allowed Del to concentrate his efforts on establishing control over different location, proximity, and people conditions. As a by-product of his success, he no longer felt panicky about panicking.

EXERCISE: USING THE CARD-SORT TECHNIQUE

Create your own card-sort ranking system to expose yourself to situations that you avoid. List location, people, or proximity conditions, ranking them from your least fearful to most fearful situations. Note that you may need to deal with only location and proximity issues or only proximity and people issues, so modify the card-sort technique as you need to.

YOUR CARD-SORT PROGRAM

Location Conditions	People Conditions	Proximity Conditions

The card-sort technique works best when you have a specific fear that you can rank in terms of least to most intense conditions.

OVERCOMING FEAR AND ANXIETY FOLLOWING TRAUMA

In his classical conditioning experiments with dogs, the famous Russian physiologist Ivan Pavlov paired a neutral stimulus, a bell, with a shock. The dog heard the bell. Within a fraction of a second, the animal also felt a shock. After several pairings, the bell evoked fear. The bell is called a conditioned stimulus. Through its close association with the shock, the bell comes to evoke fear.

When a startle-fear reaction attaches to a neutral feature of the environment, that feature becomes relevant. For example, people who suffer from post-traumatic shock often associate parts of the environment where the trauma took place with the traumatic experience.

• *Sandra's Story*

Sandra was on the third floor of a college dormitory that caught fire. She exited coughing, gasping for air, and teary eyed from the smoke. She later thought a lot about the fire and her close call. For several years after the event, Sandra felt panicky when she smelled smoke. She wouldn't go near a third floor. It got to the point where she worried her anxiety could eventually affect her health.

Ordinarily, the more you engage a conditioned stimulus in short-time intervals, the more likely your fear will weaken and be extinguished (Golkar, Bellander, and Öhman 2013). However, in Sandra's case, longer intervals were necessary. She went to a restaurant with a wood-burning fireplace and obtained a table at the farthest point from the fire. She went with her favorite friends. She ordered her favorite food. Over a two-month period, she progressively sat at tables closer and closer to the fire. Her fear of the smell of smoke dropped to nearly zero. However, she still did not like the smell of smoke.

To overcome her fear of third floors, she intentionally pushed the third and fourth floor button on an elevator. When the elevator reached the third floor, the door opened. At first, she stayed at the back of the elevator. When she felt comfortable, she moved toward the middle of the elevator. Eventually, she walked out of the elevator and then back inside before the door closed. Soon she was able to get off at the third floor without trepidation. She repeated this exposure experiment by walking down the stairs—the condition that most closely approximated what had happened in her college dorm—until she no longer felt afraid.

Should Sandra have spent time and energy dealing with panicky situations that she could normally avoid and that didn't interfere in any significant way with her life? She wanted to stop ruminating about the fire. She wanted to stop feeling afraid of safe situations. Afterward, she no longer felt panicky with the smell of smoke, she no longer felt panicky about being on a third floor, and she no longer ruminated about the fire.

In some cases, addressing one fear has a transdiagnostic effect on others. Sometimes, there is no such effect. Nevertheless, you can apply what you learned in one anxiety-fear situation to another. Judy, Del, and Sandra experienced significant fears that generalized to other areas of their lives. In addressing these primary fears, they were each able to transfer what they'd learned to other related fears. Knowing what to do, and knowing that you can do it, is advantageous!

YOUR PROGRESS REPORT

Write down what you learned from this chapter and what actions you plan to take. Then record what resulted from taking these actions and what you've gained.

What are three key ideas that you took away from this chapter?

1.

2.

3.

What top three actions can you take to combat a specific anxiety or fear?

1.

2.

3.

What resulted when you took these actions?

1.

2.

3.

What did you gain from taking action? What would you do differently next time?

1.

2.

3.

How to Address Special Anxieties and Fears

- Take a test to see where you stand on worrying.

- Learn multiple ways to stop worrying.

- Control fear of the unknown with a five-phases-of-change program.

- Overcome fear of failure.

- Build tolerance for unpleasant anxious sensations.

- See how to tone down your anxiety thinking.

- Learn what goes into a panic reaction.

- Discover how to free yourself from panic.

- Use scientifically proven ways to overcome phobias and fears.

- Use a classic method to overcome fear.

- Learn a multimodal approach to overcome anxiety.

- Discover when anxiety signals that something has gone wrong.

CHAPTER 13

Escaping a Web of Worry

Worry is a form of mental uneasiness about negative possibilities that rarely happen. It's a verbal, ruminative, language-rich process. How often do you worry in images? Probably not much!

Our ability to fret about frightening possibilities has been around for a long time. The Old English word *wyrgan* meant to choke or strangle. In the seventeenth century, the word "worry" meant to stress, trouble, or prosecute. In the nineteenth century, the word took on its current meaning: a feeling of apprehension, trouble, and unease about a possible event.

You also can view worry as repetitive negative thinking that cuts across many conditions such as phobias, panic, and social anxieties (Olatunji, Naragon-Gainey, and Wolitzky-Taylor 2013). Worry—the brooding and uncontrollable variety—is a cardinal symptom of generalized anxiety, but not all people who worry have general anxiety (Penney, Mazmanian, and Rudanycz 2013). By reducing worry, you can diminish undesirable conditions that link to it (Kertz et al. 2012).

WHAT CAUSES WORRY

A worrying habit can come from inborn tendencies toward worrying, the social models who showed you how to do it, and your own creative mind. But there is something more. You get a reward for worrying. When your dire prediction proves false, you feel relief. Relief reinforces worry.

Do you worry hardly at all or a lot? Where do you stand on the worry scale?

EXERCISE: TAKING YOUR WORRY INVENTORY

Respond to each of the statements as true or false. Check "true" if the statement applies to you or "false" if it does not.

	True	False
1. "I often think of bad things that can happen."		
2. "When a friend or family member is late, I worry about an accident."		
3. "I worry about people rejecting me."		
4. "When the phone rings, I think it will be bad news."		
5. "The world is full of harmful dangers."		
6. "I worry that people will take advantage of me."		
7. "I worry about getting into accidents."		
8. "I worry about losing my health."		
9. "I worry about contracting a fatal disease."		
10. "I worry about money."		
11. "I worry about how I look."		
12. "Climate change worries me."		
13. "I worry about not being popular."		
14. "I worry about failing."		
15. "I worry about losing my job."		
16. "I worry about dying."		
17. "I worry about looking anxious."		

If you checked "false" to every item, you probably don't worry much. If you checked "true" to most items, you probably worry a lot, and this is a problem for you. If you are somewhere in between, some worries may matter a lot while some issues barely concern you. In some instances, the numbers don't matter as much as the meaning that you place on a future possibility.

There is some good news. The ruminative, brooding nature of worry is a transdiagnostic issue. Change the process and you can break a network of related conditions. The first step is to explore whether what you are feeling is worry or anxiety.

WORRY VS. ANXIETY

Both worry and anxiety occur in the present, on a time dimension, and they often overlap each other. Although existing in the present, both relate to what is in the future.

The terms *worry* and *anxiety* have different scientific meanings, but as with the terms *anxiety* and *fear*, the meanings are often blurred. Worry is more of a negative uneasiness of the mind that relates to uncertainties and worst-case possibilities. Worry is normally made up of fictions to explain uncertainties. It is sometimes referred to as anxious apprehension. Anxiety is an emotional arousal coupled with physical signs, such as a quickened heartbeat, a change in breathing, and tightened muscles.

Worry and anxiety may share some common space in the mind and brain but also have separate places. Worry shows more left-brain activity. Worry and rumination tend to be more verbal and reflect an overactivity of the prefrontal cortex (Berkowitz et al. 2007). Anxious arousal, or anxiety, shows more right-brain activity (Engels et al. 2007). In some instances, worry serves as a distraction—avoidance—from addressing anxiety (Spielberg et al. 2013.)

The brain has many cross-connections. Worry can change to anxiety when what-if-thinking about dreaded possibilities escalates into catastrophic thinking. In a catastrophizing state of mind, you can experience an increased heart rate, sweating, and feelings of unreality. Worry can also escalate into anxiety through double troubles. As you worry about feeling anxious and losing control, you may stir up the anxious arousal that you fear to experience.

Top Tip: *When Worry Signals That Something's Wrong*

Dr. Susan Krauss Whitbourne is a professor of psychology at the University of Massachusetts in Amherst, the author of *Abnormal Psychology: Clinical Perspectives on Psychological Disorders* and *The Search for Fulfillment: Revolutionary New Research That Reveals the Secret to Long-Term Happiness*, and a regular columnist at PsychologyToday.com. She shares her perspective on worry and anxiety:

"Worry is a natural emotion that occurs when we feel threatened. However, many of our worries are unfounded and counterproductive.

"There's a natural human tendency to overestimate the dangers of taking actions that would actually help us. It seems that the brain is wired to worry first and think second.

"When we're threatened, a little structure in the limbic system called the amygdala screams out in fear, sending its signals upward to the cortex. However, the interaction between the limbic system and the cortex works in both directions. Your limbic system informs your cortex, but your cortex can also control your limbic system. It takes effort, but you can put your cortex to work to override those worry signals from the amygdala.

"Worries in daily life often take the form of subconscious, irrational ruminations over possible threats to our well-being. For example, you may worry that you'll make a terrible mistake the next time you get into a new relationship. If you let that worry dominate, you'll be so reluctant to take the plunge that you may miss out on great opportunities to meet new people.

"Sometimes it's actually good to worry, especially if there's a real danger lurking in the shadows. You should worry about losing your job if you're continually late for work or about losing your partner if you're unfaithful. In these situations, worry is a signal that something's wrong. Once you address these realistic worries by changing your behavior, you'll have no need to fret because you will have made the problem go away.

"Some may argue that the fact that we are hardwired to worry is evolutionarily based. However, what makes us distinctly human is precisely our ability to use our cortex to override the emotional storms that brew in our subcortical brain regions. By controlling your worries, you'll not only make better decisions but also feel better because you do."

ADDRESSING YOUR WORRIES

You may identify with your worry, telling yourself or others "I'm a worrier," "I'm a worrywart," or "It's my personality." When thinking about worry in this way, it is helpful to keep a fair perspective. Even if you worry a lot, there are probably many more instances where you do not make hurricanes out of passing breezes. With that in mind, you can learn how to change your worrisome thoughts to passing breezes.

Separate the Possible from the Probable

Worry involves making a magical leap from possibilities to probabilities. Remember Chicken Little, the fabled barnyard chicken who, upon feeling a stick hit its wing, panicked itself and the other animals into thinking that the sky was falling? That's what happens when we make inferences about what's possible and then fret over what probably won't happen.

It's true that anything is possible. However, would you bet your life's income on your current prophecy coming true? If you wouldn't, here is an exercise for you.

EXERCISE: SEPARATING THE POSSIBLE FROM THE PROBABLE

In the left column, list your worries, or what you are afraid will happen. In the right column, estimate the probability of these worries being realized. What is the probability that each of these events will happen? You can estimate probability on a scale of 0 to 100, where 0 means there is no chance it will happen and 100 means it will happen with 100 percent certainty.

Possibility Worries	Probability Examination

If you flip a coin, it's nearly 100 percent certain that it will come up either heads or tails. It's highly unlikely the coin will land on its edge. Unlike a coin toss, where the odds are known, it's highly improbable that your recurring worries will always and accurately predict the events that consume your attention.

Recurring worries are driven by psychological factors, including magical beliefs that by worrying you can avert disaster. Rather than let these ruminations go unchecked, use the previous exercise to stop jumping to conclusions about remote possibilities. You may worry less.

Examine Your Worry Speculations

People who routinely worry may make a case to support their worries by supporting them with specious evidence. For example, your boss appears indifferent, and you take your boss's demeanor to mean you could lose your job. You then weave together bits and pieces of information that support your worry. For example, you heard that because the economy is slowing, your company will have to cut back on its workforce. It's all very clear. You worry that you will be severed from your job by the end of the day. The following day, you repeat a similar cycle of worry. In an odd way, this worry is like a superstition that protects you from an outcome that you fear.

A river cluttered with debris that dams the water's flow has limited use. In a sense, this is like a mind filled with the clutter of ungrounded worrisome speculations and assumptions that, when woven together, impede the flow of productive thought. Whenever you are tangled in worry, a first line of defense is to think about your thinking and separate speculation from fact.

EXERCISE: EXAMINING YOUR WORRY SPECULATIONS

In the left column, list your worry speculations. Then in the right column, give evidence to support them. You may have trouble proving a speculation and may feel forced to conclude that your worry speculations are more specious than factual. This is your reality examination.

Worry Speculations	Reality Examination

You can learn to stop making a case in support of your worries. All it takes is recognizing and examining speculative thoughts. When you put worry in perspective, you are free to address the objects of your anxiety.

Break the Could-Be-Thinking Trap

Practically anything could happen. A comet could hit you. Will it happen today? It could! In a long-running TV comedy series, *Monk*, a genius crime solver is portrayed as a consummate worrier. The show's theme song, "It's a Jungle Out There," captures the essence of Monk's plight. For Monk, there is chaos everywhere and poison is in the air. Bad things could happen, and Monk is painfully aware of what they are.

Monk's overly cautious approach to everyday activities made him a lovable character. A sub-group of viewers could truly understand his excessive fear of snakes, worries about contaminants in the air, heights, milk, and other aspects of normal daily living. After all, you could encounter a snake. You could drink contaminated milk. To overcome this kind of thinking, you have to ask yourself, will it really happen? The answer is probably not.

For his part, Monk couldn't be convinced that his obsessive fears were extreme. That's because his worries were a defense against an inner pain following a major loss. He couldn't control the loss. But he could control the water he drank. He could stay away from high places.

When unlikely possibilities translate into worry feelings, you've created a certainty out of a fiction. You'll then fill in the gaps to support the worry. This kind of thinking can be a habit, a defense, or both a habit and a defense. If you find yourself in such *could-be-thinking* traps, figure out what is going on.

EXERCISE: EXAMINING COULD-BE-THINKING

In the left column, write down your could-be-thinking worry talk. In the right column, do a reality review.

"Could Be" Worry Talk	"Could Be" Reality Review

The old adage "Don't sweat the small stuff" takes on a new meaning when worrisome small stuff detracts from the big stuff, or what you are putting off in your life that's really important to you. However, there are many other ways to create a crisis, including ballooning something fictional into something big.

Contend with the If-Then-Thinking Trap

Some people have many *if-then-thinking* worries. More often than not, if-then-thinking balloons a possibility into a crisis. Here's an example of this kind of worry: "If John doesn't call in the next five minutes, then he has gotten into an accident." The trick is to recognize the "if" and the "then" in this worry cycle, and then to impose reason between the premise and the conclusion.

A misguided major premise (if John doesn't call), followed by an erroneous secondary premise (five minutes is the standard), can become the foundation for a speculative conclusion (John got in an accident). You can neutralize these thought associations by interjecting the question, "If not, then what?" Five minutes pass, and you don't hear from John, so you think, "If it's not an accident, then what?" You might consider that the battery went dead or that John has been delayed by another phone call.

EXERCISE: DISMANTLING IF-THEN-THINKING TRAPS

In the left column, write down some examples of what you tell yourself might happen with if-then worry talk. In the right column, consider the "If not, then what?" question. For example, if what you fear most won't happen, what benign event could happen instead?

If-Then Worry Talk	"If Not, Then What?"

Examining your worry thinking by asking "If not, then what?" will help you undo this thinking trap. As an alternative, devising strategies to cope with remote possibilities may make you feel better, but you may soon discover that you spend a lot of time planning solutions for disasters that never happen.

Top Tip: Take One Step at a Time

Dr. Pamela D. Garcy, a clinical psychologist in Dallas, author of *The REBT Super-Activity Guide*, and webmaster at Myinnerguide.com, shares how to eliminate worry, one step at a time:

"Here are four tips for helping yourself eliminate worry:

1. When you catch yourself worrying, ask yourself, 'Is there someone who can help me with my situation?' Making a request may help you to set a limit or gain helpful support, thereby reducing worrying.

2. Take a helpful action step, however small. Taking almost any positive action step to improve your situation will empower you and reduce your worrying.

3. Sometimes people have too many actions steps to do. If you fall into this trap, ask yourself, 'What's next?' Focus only on this one thing. Breathe slowly in and out as you go. When you complete this action, reward yourself with a short break and then ask, 'What's next?'

4. Still stuck? Try a focus-changing technique. Start by making a table with two columns. At the top of the table, write out what you're worrying about. In the first column, write out everything that is out of your control about the situation (such as another person's behavior, another's opinion, or what someone else says). At the bottom of this column, write down how you feel when you focus upon the aspects of the problem that are out of your control. In the second column, write down everything that is in your control about the situation (such as how you think, what you say or don't say, or whether or not you act in one way or another). At the bottom of this column, write down how you feel when you focus upon the aspects of the problem that are in your control. This will help you to gain clarity about what you can do and where you want to place your emphasis."

Dodge the Theory Trap

Worries are like theories: you can make them sound reasonable and then think they must be true. But a theory is not the same as a fact.

For centuries, our ancestors thought the world was flat. Operating on this theory, sailing ships tended to go along known sea paths or within sight of shore to avoid falling off the face of the earth. There was practical value to this thinking fallacy. By sticking to known shipping channels, you were less likely to get lost at sea. However, believing that the world is flat doesn't change the reality that the earth is spherical.

To dodge the trap of treating your worry theories as facts, look for ways to support the opposite theory. If you theorize that a rogue asteroid will hit the earth in six months, flip the theory. Ask yourself what facts support that conclusion.

EXERCISE: EVALUATING WORRY THEORIES

In the left column, write down a theory of yours that causes worry. In the right column, write down some facts that support the opposite theory.

Worry Theory	Worry Theory Examination

What do you conclude from this examination?

A few other techniques for addressing worry are worth testing.

General Techniques for Defeating Worry

You can add several more practical techniques to your quiver of methods to address worry thinking:

Group your worries. By dividing your worries into two different groups, what you can do something about and what you can't do anything about, you can dismantle this thinking trap. If you can't do anything about a possible outcome, why worry? If you can do something about it, then devise a coping strategy.

Nip worry in the bud by naming the process. Start by describing worry as automatic verbal ruminations that kick up emotional dust. Labeling worry in this way can help put this thought pattern into perspective.

Plot a mindfulness course. This can be as simple as thinking about a worrisome thought running on a treadmill and getting nowhere. Such changes in thinking responses to anxiety are associated with reductions in worry (Querstret and Cropley 2013).

Ask the simple question "Do I feel like continuing?" This question implies that if worry thinking is no longer enjoyable or profitable, you can terminate it (Davey et al. 2007).

Separate concern from worry. When you have concern for yourself, someone else, or a situation, you care about what is happening. Because you care, you want to act responsibly. Next time you worry, ask yourself, "How can I act responsibly about worry?"

Flip perspectives. Say a friend is late and you start to worry. You don't know what's happening. You can't control what you don't know. So ask yourself, if you were late and knew what was happening, would you want someone else to worry about you? If not, why not?

Play with paradoxes. Daily, schedule ten minutes of time to worry. At that time, think about what you have to worry about. Under controlled worry conditions, you may find your mind drifting from the worries.

Wear an elastic band on your wrist. When you start to worry, snap the elastic band. Do it hard enough to be uncomfortable without breaking the skin. Instead of being rewarded for worry, you thus experience this immediate mild punishment. You could also use a thought-stopping technique. When you start to worry, silently shout, *Stop, stop, stop!* in your mind.

Give the word "worry" a new meaning. Use it as an acronym to stand for these corrective actions: *Will* yourself to act against worry. *Organize* to address worries; test your plan whenever you are caught off guard. *Reflect* productively by separating facts from fiction. *Respond* with active measures to control what you can and to accept what you can't. *Yield* to the reality that worries will recur; you don't have to take them seriously.

Top Tip: How to Stop Dutifully Worrying

Dr. Elliot D. Cohen, president of the Institute of Critical Thinking: National Center for Logic-Based Therapy, and author of *The Dutiful Worrier*, shares some valuable pointers for defusing worries and anxiety:

"One kind of anxiety that involves chronic worry and rumination is what I have called 'dutiful worrying.' The dutiful worrier worries and ruminates about problems she perceives to portend catastrophic consequences. She tells herself that if she does not worry about the perceived problem at hand, then the perceived catastrophic consequences will occur; it will be her fault; she will be a bad person for letting these terrible things happen; and that, therefore, she has a moral duty to worry about the perceived problem until she finds a perfect (or near perfect) solution to it. Because there are no perfect solutions, the dutiful worrier persists in ruminating about the 'crisis' until it is 'resolved,' often by indecision, and then the focus shifts to a new worry, and the vicious cycle continues.

"Here are a few constructive pointers in rationally confronting this kind of anxiety. First, most things that you worry about are not likely to have catastrophic consequences. Thus, ask yourself what evidence you have to justify your belief that such consequences will happen.

Second, you cannot control everything, so you should stick to addressing what you can control, which includes how you think about things but not external events, such as other people's actions, economic conditions, the existence of evil in the world, and so forth. Third, you should accept the veritable fact that the world is imperfect and that there is therefore no perfect solution to the problems of living. Fourth, it is unreasonable to demand certainty in making your decisions, so you should live by probabilities, not certainties. Fifth, you do not have a moral duty to worry. In fact, worrying and ruminating do not solve problems; instead they defeat your ability to act proactively in addressing your problems. Sixth, when you do have a real problem (one for which you do have adequate evidence), you should act proactively to resolve it. Devise a plan of action and stick to it. Worry and rumination just get in the way of resolving your problems of living."

YOUR PROGRESS REPORT

Write down what you learned from this chapter and what actions you plan to take. Then record what resulted from taking these actions and what you've gained.

What are three key ideas that you took away from this chapter?

1.

2.

3.

What top three actions can you take to combat a specific anxiety or fear?

1.

2.

3.

What resulted when you took these actions?

1.

2.

3.

What did you gain from taking action? What would you do differently next time?

1.

2.

3.

CHAPTER 14

Managing Anxiety over Uncertainty

When you feel threatened and anxious, security is important and change is disruptive. With this mind-set, you may believe that you dare not stray from familiar paths. The truth is that planned deviations could be an antidote to your anxieties over uncertainties, but you also don't know for sure what will happen if you try. As a result, you may make special efforts to keep things predictable.

INTOLERANCE FOR UNCERTAINTY

Anxiety about uncertainty worsens anxiety (Dugas et al. 2007). Faced with uncertainty and with a need for predictability, you can feel paralyzed (Birrella et al. 2011). With an intolerance for uncertainty, you are likely to worry excessively (Buhr and Dugas 2006). Worry, then, is like a double-edged sword. You feel held back by the weight of worry, and you worry because you feel held back. You stay put because you have no guarantees that you can bring about the sort of changes in your life that can break this cycle.

Intolerance for uncertainty is a transdiagnostic factor that cuts across generalized anxiety, social anxiety, depression, panic, agoraphobia, and ruminations, among other conditions (Mahoney and McEvoy 2012). CBT methods that apply to creating control over uncertainty are related to progress in overcoming anxiety (Gallagher, Naragon-Gainey, and Brown 2014).

If only you had a guarantee that your efforts would be productive, you'd stray from the protective paths that you typically follow. Unfortunately, there are no guarantees. However, you can roll the dice in favor of less anxiety and greater well-being when you take steps associated with gaining clarity by making positive changes.

FIVE STEPS TO FREEDOM FROM ANXIETY OVER UNCERTAINTY

You can overcome anxieties about uncertainties using my five-phases-of-change approach: awareness, action, accommodation, acceptance, and actualization.

Awareness

If you think you have more than your share of anxieties and fears, you may be reluctant to risk feeling even greater tension by engaging what you fear, especially if you are unsure of what to expect. Indeed, the thought of change—even a positive one—can stir up doubts that you can handle any more tension. However, building greater awareness is a critical first step in the process of making positive voluntary changes.

What is this phase in the process of change that we call "awareness"? It means engaging your consciousness about what is taking place within and around you. It involves knowing the makeup of your anxieties and what you can realistically do to overcome them. By testing your growing knowledge and resources, you increase your awareness even further as you develop into a stronger, more confident you. As an example, a client whose anxiety was chiefly triggered by social situations filled out this questionnaire.

Awareness-of-Uncertainty Questionnaire

Awareness-Building Questions	Awareness-Building Answers
1. What situations trigger your anxious thoughts and feelings about uncertainty?	*Practically any social situation where there is no guarantee that I can control the outcome: speaking before a group, joining a club, attending a wedding.*
2. When you experience intolerance for uncertainty, what do you normally do?	*Worry. Give up. Make up excuses. Avoid the occasion.*
3. What conditions amplify your risk for intolerance for uncertainty? Ambiguous circumstances? Mood? Conflicts? Finances? Health?	*Being overweight and lack of exercise do it for me. Unexpected inconveniences, such as my car breaking down, an overdue water bill, gloomy weather. Drinking too much at times.*

4. What cognitions, emotions, and behaviors do you associate with intolerance for uncertainty?	Cognitions: *Change is too risky. Can fail. Can look awkward. Will embarrass self. Will fail. Worry that I will never get over these feelings.* Emotions: *Anxiety. Irritation. Anger at times. Depressed.* Behaviors: *Eat, drink, and smoke to calm nerves.*
5. What increases your anxieties about uncertainties? What decreases them?	Increases: *Fatigue. Lack of sleep. Wintertime. Boring job.* Decreases: *Exercise. Sleeping well. Doing something to address anxieties: challenging worry talk.*
6. What are the consequences of living with intolerance for uncertainty?	*Have abilities and a college degree, but take low-level repetitive jobs. Quality work is missing. Vehicle is a clunker; prefer a new car. Lacking feeling of stability and self-worth.*
7. What works best for you to combat your intolerance for uncertainty?	*Sit back, reflect, figure out what to do, and then try to do it. But some things happen fast and take quick decisions. Mostly retreat, but when trying to sort things out on the spot, can sometimes work "miracles." Avoiding hesitations and delays seems to help. It's the anticipation of something awful about to happen that feels crushing.*

EXERCISE: BUILDING AWARENESS OF UNCERTAINTY

Answer these questions to chart what goes into your intolerance for uncertainty and to bring clarity to your situation.

Your Awareness-of-Uncertainty Questionnaire

Awareness-Building Questions	Awareness-Building Answers
1. What situations trigger your anxious thoughts and feelings about uncertainty?	
2. When you experience intolerance for uncertainty, what do you normally do?	
3. What conditions amplify your risk for intolerance for uncertainty? Ambiguous circumstances? Mood? Conflicts? Finances? Health?	
4. What cognitions, emotions, and behaviors do you associate with intolerance for uncertainty?	Cognitions: Emotions: Behaviors:
5. What increases your anxieties about uncertainties? What decreases them?	Increases: Decreases:
6. What are the consequences of living with intolerance for uncertainty?	
7. What works best for you to combat your intolerance for uncertainty?	

Now that you know what works best for you, why not do what you know works?

Action

To change, you have to do something different. If you want to cross the street in a different way, you'll have to take new steps. If you want to build self-confidence, you'll have to start thinking and acting like a self-confident person.

Action is the process of taking steps to achieve the goal of ridding yourself of burdensome anxieties and fears. Thus, if you feel anxious about uncertainty, you'd be wise to enter that zone of uncertainty for the greater purpose of obtaining clarity and direction. Clarity born from experience adds a dose of realism to awareness.

Encountering Fear of Failure

When you have gaps in your knowledge, you necessarily have uncertainty. By entering situations with imperfect information, you could fail, which may stop you from going any further. But what would it mean if you took a learn-as-you-go approach? What if you could eliminate the specter of failure when it comes to engaging in self-development activities?

A Scientific Approach to Fear of Failure

A scientific pursuit is a nonjudgmental process of discovery. A scientist sets up hypotheses, or propositions, and tests them to see what happens. If you follow this process, you can't fail in your self-improvement efforts. Rather, you see what works, what doesn't, and where you still have work to do.

As with any useful scientific study, you would start this one with a question: "What actions do I take to get past this uncertainty barrier to change?" You could then generate cognitive, emotive, and behavioral hypotheses:

Hypothesis 1: *All reasons for intolerance for uncertainty are valid.* Examine this hypothesis to see if you can falsify it. Instead of looking to prove that your fear of uncertainty reflects real threats, find ways to poke holes in your anxiety thinking.

Hypothesis 2: *It's impossible to build emotional tolerance for uncertainty.* Test this hypothesis by acting to substitute emotional tolerance for the intolerance of uncertainty. First allow yourself to feel the feeling of anxiety, but in a different way. Isolate the location of the tension sensations. Mark their locations (for example, stomach, shoulders, neck). Isolating areas of tension is a step in the direction of tolerating anxiety. By isolating tension zones, you open new options. For example, you can accept each as a symptom of tension. This acceptance—along with relaxing each tension zone—can reduce the physical effects of anxiety.

Hypothesis 3: *Facing conditions of uncertainty is a formula for resolving situations that you associate with distress.* To test this proposition, enter your region of uncertainty to determine if you can find answers, make discoveries, and develop tolerance.

EXERCISE: TURNING FEAR OF FAILURE INTO HYPOTHESES

Involve yourself in a behavioral process to reduce uncertainty by testing hypotheses and new behaviors. Answer the following questions:

1. What uncertainty do you want to resolve?

2. What's your motivation (benefit)?

3. Cite the hypothesis that you will test.

4. Describe how you will test the hypothesis.

5. What did you discover about uncertainty from taking these steps?

Few things in life go as smoothly as we hope or as badly as we might expect. Undertakings that include uncertainties—even those with reasonable positive expectancies—can have unexpected complications or result in happy accidents. Expect variations and fluctuations in life and you won't be disappointed.

Accommodation

Accommodation means adjusting to new ways of thinking and acting. For you, accommodation might mean reconciling conflicting thoughts, say, about an intolerance toward uncertainty, and the reality that life is filled with ambiguities.

This is an intellectual-integration phase of change, where you put your anxiety over uncertainty into perspective. By placing yourself in conditions of uncertainty, you can come to know the problem better, and this awareness can reduce uncertainty. You'll often find that what you feared wasn't as bad as you expected it to be. If what you hope to happen doesn't pan out, you can make adjustments in your thinking and actions.

Our inner struggles frequently involve conflicts between our negative and positive self-views. We have conflicts between anxiety and self-mastery, doubts and self-command, certainty and uncertainty. Through accommodation thinking, you can see which has the greater validity. Suppose you think poorly of yourself and feel anxious because you believe that others think as badly of you as you do of yourself. Yet you routinely receive positive feedback from others. How do you reconcile this difference? Perhaps part of the answer lies in recognizing that you can change unwanted parts of your thoughts, feelings, and actions, even if changing is difficult and you have no guarantees."

How do you resolve this disparity between what you think of yourself and what others are telling you? If you cling to negative information that you believe about yourself, then you are resolving uncertainty by confirming a negative self-view. If you take positive new feedback into account, then you are accommodating to positive feedback about yourself.

Examining disparities between anxiety beliefs and observations that contradict those beliefs can prompt conflict, and conflict correlates with an unpleasant feeling of tension.

But how bad is the feeling of tension? Can you accommodate it? Would you accept $10,000 a day for living with one hour of tension as you sought ways to resolve a conflict between an old anxiety-ridden self-view and an adaptive new self-view? You might if you believed that tension over uncertainty is a time-limited experience. And it is!

You may believe that you are helpless to change your anxieties about uncertainties even though you have evidence that you can make voluntary changes. How do you reconcile this incongruity? Perhaps the answer is to recognize that you can change unwanted parts of your thoughts, feelings, and actions even if changing is difficult.

Creating an Accommodating Attitude

Your anxiety may increase when you think seriously about what might happen as you start to address your anxieties and fears. True, there are many uncertainties. You may not be sure of where to begin. You could feel awkward and self-conscious as you start to experiment. But this is where you want to be—at the precipice of clarity.

To create a more accommodating attitude, you can redirect your thinking toward the benefits of solving fear-related problems and reducing uncertainties. A short- and long-term benefits analysis is a classic way to gain perspective on this issue. In this exercise, you compare the short-term benefits of repeating anxiety cycles with the long-term benefits of living through the discomfort of working through your anxieties and their sibling fears:

Course of Action	Short-Term Benefits	Long-Term Benefits
Do nothing formal to change anxiety for uncertainty.	Avoid immediate discomfort. Experience relief from worry when feared events don't happen.	Avoid immediate discomfort. Experience relief from worry when feared events don't happen.

Challenge anxiety over uncertainty.	Begin to see that constructive actions lead to clarity and the sort of relief that follows taking charge of your life.	A coping self-efficacy perspective. Reduction in anxieties and fear about uncertainty. Acting on more opportunities. Decreased frequency, intensity, and duration of anxieties and fears about uncertainty. Increased ability to handle inconvenience. Improved problem-solving skills. Less stress on the body.

By doing a benefits analysis, you can see how the results of challenging anxiety about uncertainty differ from the results of maintaining your anxiety. Now you can do your own benefits analysis.

EXERCISE: YOUR BENEFITS ANALYSIS

Write down the benefits for maintaining anxiety of uncertainty and the benefits for challenging this anxiety. Do the benefits of challenging anxiety of uncertainty outweigh the benefits for maintaining it?

Course of Action	Short-Term Benefits	Long-Term Benefits
Do nothing formal to change anxiety of uncertainty.		
Challenge anxiety over uncertainty.		

Although you may not relish approaching uncertain circumstances, feeling free to engage them is a far better position than dodging uncertainty because of excessive wariness and fear of the feeling of anxiety.

Acceptance

The next step is acceptance, which involves emotional integration. The spirit of acceptance is that of resigning yourself to outside realities that are not going to change. For example, you would acknowledge that rivers sometimes flood or recognize that you can have different political views from your cousin. At the same time, you don't have to like the fact that rivers flood, especially if a flooding river swept your house away. You may not like your cousin's political perspective. But such things are as they are.

There can be many things that you'd like to control but can't, and you need not distress yourself over such matters. Knowing that you can't control the speed of the sun is unlikely to bother you. However, in situations where control can make a difference, and that control is in doubt, the picture can change. You may want your neighbor to live according to rules you find worthwhile, such as keeping her dog off of your lawn, but your neighbor doesn't have the same beliefs as you. In this case, acceptance doesn't mean that you are stymied. You could ask your neighbor to keep her dog off your lawn. You could put up a fence.

When you look back over your life, you will find good times and bad times and many in-between times. Some of life's events will truly be regrettable, and it's impossible to do anything to change what has happened. You have the choice of acceptance. Now what about acceptance of what is happening in the present?

Acceptance doesn't mean you are passively bound to a turnstile. In an acceptant state of mind, you can do the following:

- See events as having potential for evoking different perspectives.

- See events for what they are and not as what you would like them to be.

- Acknowledge what is going on within and around you.

- Make mental adjustments to tolerate discomfort, disappointment, fear, and frustration.

In an acceptant state of mind, you focus on what you can develop, improve, cope with, change, or accomplish. In short, if you don't like a situation, you can take action to effect a change. If you can't change a negative situation that is already in process, you find a way to adjust.

Not everything in the present moment or future is clear. Ambiguity and uncertainty are a part of the present and future. But you can work on incorporating these five points of uncertainty into your life:

- Accept facts and reality.

- Accept that you can progressively master methods for overcoming uncertainty fears.

- Accept that a prime solution to overcoming anxiety involves experiencing uncertainty fears at the time and in the space in which they occur.

- Accept that preparing for uncertainty may prove uncomfortable but is instrumental to positive change.

- Accept that overpreparation, such as repeatedly going over every possible scenario, supports a misguided view that perfection is the solution for controlling tension.

Top Tip: Life Is Uncertain. Deal with It.

Dr. John Minor is an associate fellow and training faculty member in REBT. This University of California adjunct professor shares a tip for controlling an intolerance for uncertainty that can catapult into an extreme anxiety:

"Anxiety can feel intense when you face uncertainties about the future and when you believe that you won't be able to handle whatever hidden threat is in store for you. It's helpful to recognize and unashamedly acknowledge anxiety proneness under conditions of uncertainty. You'll be less likely to suffer the pangs of intolerance toward uncertainty and intolerance for anxiety.

"To actively cope with an intolerance for uncertainty, first make a list of your (conscious) areas where uncertainty is a catalyst for anxiety. Then rate the items on your list from 1 to 10, where 1 means little or no anxiety and 10 means extreme dread or terror. Did any seem worse than 10, or 'too awful' to rate (worse than 100 percent bad)? Now imagine something even worse than the worst. If you can do that, it means that situations with a 100 percent-plus rating aren't totally bad. By routinely doing this rating, you will hopefully see that awfulizing over uncertainty is an exaggeration. Exaggerations can be replaced by rational views, such as 'Uncertainty in life is a proven fact. I want to tolerate it as well as I can. I want to be more rational. I prefer calmness to anxiety. I can stand my anxiety about future uncertainties.'"

Actualization

Actualization means stretching your abilities to discover what you can do in areas that are important to you. Instead of absorbing yourself in worries and troubles over uncertainties, you absorb yourself in what you are doing. In that way, you learn more about what you can accomplish.

A prime actualization objective is to decrease negatives by striving for positive results. As you move in this direction, you no longer avoid uncertainties just because they stir discomfort. By striking out in a positive direction, you reach beyond your uncertainties. You move toward gaining clarity and making gains. You feel much more in command of yourself and in charge of your life.

EXERCISE: START ACTUALIZING

Articulate the steps you need to take to move yourself forward on an enlightened pathway toward what you'd truly like to accomplish. Write down your goal for pushing past uncertainty to meet vital challenges, describe the short- and long-term benefits of achieving this goal, and then outline what you will do to achieve it.

1. What do you want to accomplish?

2. What are the short- and long-term benefits of pursuing this goal?

3. Outline what you can and will do to address anxiety over uncertainty as you stretch for your goal.

Now begin executing the steps to gain freedom over uncertainty.

With awareness, action, accommodation, acceptance, and actualization, you can increase your tolerance for anxiety from uncertainty. It's not even necessary to follow the steps in this exact order. Voluntary personal change doesn't have to follow a specific sequence. You may develop new ideas and insights from the results of your actions. You may experience a radical shift in your views through accommodation. By stretching your resources, you can favorably influence the other stages in this process.

YOUR PROGRESS REPORT

Write down what you learned from this chapter and what actions you plan to take. Then record what resulted from taking these actions and what you've gained.

What are three key ideas that you took away from this chapter?

1.

2.

3.

What top three actions can you take to combat a specific anxiety or fear?

1.

2.

3.

What resulted when you took these actions?

1.

2.

3.

What did you gain from taking action? What would you do differently next time?

1.

2.

3.

CHAPTER 15

Calming Anxiety Sensations

Slight but sudden physical changes can trigger negative thoughts. These changes include sweating, an uptick in your heartbeat, increases in your breathing pattern, or muscular tension. If you associate such physical sensations with negative consequences, such as looking like a nervous wreck in front of others, this sensation detection, magnification, and interpretation process reflects an anxiety sensitivity (Reiss and McNally 1985). This anxiety sensitivity—what you think about your sensations—increases your risk for various forms of anxiety (Mantar, Yemez, and Alkin 2011).

There is no end to how far people will go to avoid unexplained and unpleasant sensations. While at a shopping mall, a client named Don felt dizzy and had a quickened heart rate. He felt so anxious about this happening again that he went on Valium and stayed on it even though the medication fogged his mind, sapped his energy, and increased his anxiety. When he did feel good, Don tried so hard to cling to feeling good that he felt tense.

Ducking and hiding from unpleasant sensations rarely turns out well. Psychiatrist Abraham Low (1950) points out that the more you anticipate the discomfort you fear, the greater the fear that you will feel. Your fear of the feelings of anxiety and fear sensations can be so great that you'll repeat a cycle of sensing tension, magnifying the tension (with helpless thoughts), and scrambling to avoid unpleasant feelings. There must be a better way.

Top Tip: Make It Better by Making It Worse

Dr. Sam Klarreich is president of the Berkeley Centre for Effectiveness in Toronto and the author of eight books, including *Pressure Proofing: How to Increase Personal Effectiveness on the Job and Anywhere for That Matter*. He shares his top tip:

"When in the midst of a panic reaction, take note of all the symptoms that you are experiencing. That may be hard to do right then and there, but try your best. Pay attention to your bodily sensations and your emotional reactions. Now that you have noted these symptoms, try really hard to double the intensity of these symptoms.

"The key is to realize and truly believe that these symptoms will not hurt you, are temporary in nature, and will pass. Knowing that, you will find that as you try to double the intensity of your anxiety symptoms, they will paradoxically lessen in intensity. First, you are now facing these symptoms head on and not running in fear of them. Second, because you are facing them directly, and find that you are unable to increase their intensity, you will actually discover that they diminish."

WHAT YOU TELL YOURSELF CAN MAKE A DIFFERENCE

As if by instinct, you may seek a cause to explain your unexplained negative feelings and sensations. You scan your environment. You see a cluttered kitchen. Your mate is a slob. That's the reason. Or perhaps it's your ungrateful boss. You work hard and don't get the credit that you deserve. That's the reason.

It may be true that your mate isn't tidy or that your boss is unappreciative. But if such matters were not a hot issue yesterday or the day before, and nothing significant has changed, then why make them an issue now? Can you rule out that you feel irritable because the weather is about to change? Does your irritability have something to do with the time of the day? Did you have too much caffeine?

A Theory of Labeling

Psychologists Stanley Schachter and Jerome Singer (1962) thought that physical sensations and a cognitive label together describe an emotion. That is, when you become aroused, you'll tend to look for reasons to explain what is going on, and you may use an emotional label to explain the feeling.

Schachter and Singer's theory of emotions is imperfect, because you can have a sensation or emotion without labeling it. For example, infants don't label their emotions. However, when you come to an age where you can interpret experience by using analytic skills and language, your world changes. You may look for causes and apply labels to unexplained sensations. Depending on the context, the same sensation may be labeled anger, happiness, or fear. The label becomes your reality.

Toning Down Your Language

If you tend to go into alarm mode over negative somatic changes, you can learn to describe how you feel without dramatizing the meaning of the sensation. Milder affective labels can trickle down from the prefrontal cortex to the amygdala to help tone down negative emotional images (Lieberman et al. 2007).

You can substitute accurate but milder emotional words for dramatic language. Words like "unpleasant" or "uncomfortable" convey a different message from alarmist words like "awful" or "horrible." The phrase "I don't like feeling anxious" has a different meaning from "I can't stand feeling anxious." By toning down your language, you can avoid viewing yourself as distressed and overwhelmed.

Coping with Discomfort Fears

A *discomfort fear* is an exaggerated threat to your emotional stability (Knaus 1982). If you feel an unpleasant sensation, believe that you can't bear feeling tense, and then see yourself as emotionally falling to pieces, you have put yourself in a perilous position. But have you perhaps exaggerated the threat?

When you fall into a tension-escalating language trap, you can use affective labeling techniques to change the picture. Instead of thinking *I cannot stand discomfort*, you can redefine the problem as *I prefer not to have the discomfort, but it is what it is*.

You can make learning to tolerate tension part of engaging in a useful but uncomfortable situation. By showing yourself that you can stand tension, you are less likely to rocket normal tensions into negative emotions that you may later describe as terrible. As a bonus, you may lower your risk of overreacting to negative physical sensations and thus be less *sensation sensitive* about normal physical fluctuations. As a bonus, you may decrease secondary procrastination.

Top Tip: Slow Down, Dig In, and Live the Big Picture

Multimodal therapist Dr. Jeffrey A. Rudolph is a licensed clinical psychologist who practices in Manhattan and Ridgewood, New Jersey. Rudolph shares this tip that he uses with his clients:

"Anxiety is rooted in the false perception of threat and loss of control, muting your natural need to feel challenged and masterful. Unfortunately, many of us who view ourselves as sensitive by nature are prone to be seduced by it, getting stuck in the moment and trapped by the discomfort it elicits.

"Anxiety speeds you up. When you speed up, you lose perspective. This fuels your tendency to rush through experiences, leaving you feeling drained. Thus, dodging your anxieties can lead to seeing your cup of experiences as depleted, or half empty. Avoid lamenting lost opportunities. Remind yourself that whether your glass is half empty or half full, what is most important is the quality of the contents inside.

Here are two steps to add quality content to the mix:

1. Down shift to first gear, catch your breath, and take a moment to break down what feels overwhelming into distinct 'smaller pieces.' You are now employing what you already have—your natural ability for perspective, reasoning, and problem solving.

2. Follow my *10/40 rule*: it takes just 10 percent of purposeful effort, or a 10 percent reduction of a threatening situation, to produce a 40 percent drop in your anxiety. Apply that rule to meeting a challenge that includes getting past an anxiety that is in your way."

APPLYING OCCAM'S RAZOR

Fourteenth century philosopher William of Occam argued that the simplest explanation is probably more accurate than a more complex one. Using the principle of Occam's razor, you can trim away faulty assumptions about your uncomfortable sensations.

Physical sensations need not be scary if you read them correctly. A sudden change in how you physically feel may have a simple explanation: lower blood sugar; you are coming down with a cold; you've lost sleep; the weather is about to change. How are you to know which of the above—if any—is relevant? You may not, and that's the point. If you don't know, why speculate?

The simplest explanation is not always the correct one. Nevertheless, in combatting anxieties and fears that are fueled by elaborate evaluations and complications, shaving off the excesses can boil the problem down to its essentials.

Occam's Razor Applied to Fear-Arousing Cognitions

Sensation Complicating Evaluations	Simplest Explanations
Thoughts and feelings of terror following a jump in heart rate	Chances are your heartbeats are within exercise limits.

A quick change in your heartbeat invites explanations that can trigger fear thinking.

Over any given week, some fluctuations in breathing, heart rate, or blood pressure are normal.

The sensations feel unpleasant, but that's the only problem. |
| *I don't know what is happening. I don't know what to do. I'm helpless.* | Labeling this thinking "uncertainty thinking," "powerlessness thinking," or "fear of the unknown:" gives you target cognitions to address. Address your evaluations by asking *what* questions: "What do I factually know about what's happening? What do I know about the cognition that I associate with this fear? What coping options are open to me?" Asking and answering these clarifying questions is like taking a razor to emotion-escalating evaluations and elaborations. |
| *I'm going to spin out of control. I'm going to lose my mind. This will not stop.* | The simplest explanation is that you are catastrophizing. Label it and boil down the issue to a few basics: What does it mean to spin out of control? How can feeling fear cause you to lose your mind? If you did lose your mind, what would that be like? How could you find your mind if you lost it?

Ask yourself, where is the proof that the tension will go on forever? |

To end this review, consider that tension means you are alive and are surviving.

EXERCISE: USING OCCAM'S RAZOR

Use Occam's razor to shave off excess meaning that you know—or suspect—is bunk. Pick a physical sensation that typically causes you anxiety, write down your fear-arousing cognitions associated with the sensation, and come up with simpler explanations for what is happening.

Sensation Complicating Evaluations	Simplest Explanations
1.	
2.	
3.	

Of course, simple is not always the same as easy. Nineteenth century Prussian general Carl Von Clausewitz (1982) observed that we can make simple actions difficult by burdening ourselves with misgivings, complications, and meaningless fears. He thought that while preparation was important, action was preferable to theoretical contemplation about the uncertainties and ambiguities of situations.

LOW FRUSTRATION TOLERANCE AND DISTRESS

If you suffer from anxieties and fears about how you feel, you are likely to have a *low frustration tolerance* (LFT) for feeling tense. As a result, you may automatically avoid combatting unhealthy fears, thus perpetuating them. LFT is abetted by tension-amplifying thinking, where your words exaggerate the meaning of the tension.

Building Frustration Tolerance

High frustration tolerance and low stress are related (Mahon et al. 2007). So how can you make the shift to greater stress tolerance?

From a mindfulness-based lens, you can view LFT thinking as you might watch clouds float by. You can't control the direction of the clouds, so why upset yourself over what you can't control? Is it possible for you to let it be?

If you can't let it be, then what? You can actively question and change dramatized thinking that escalates anxiety.

Dramatized distress thinking includes such beliefs as *These feelings are too much for me to take* and *I can't cope.* This verbal chatter is like taking an uncomfortable feeling and twisting it into a major upset. Here are some examples of LFT distress beliefs, six questions you could ask to challenge this thinking, and sample answers showing how to remedy this LFT thinking process:

Questioning Dramatized Thinking

LFT Distress Beliefs	Sample Questions	Sample Answers
These feelings are too much for me to manage.	What makes that so?	*My belief. Fortunately, beliefs of this sort can be changed. For example, I can realistically say that I'd prefer to feel calm, but if I don't, tough! Life goes on.*
I can't cope.	What makes you think you can't find a way to cope?	*Even under the worst of circumstances, I can do something that gives me a chance. What is it?*
I can't stand feeling tense.	If you believe you can't stand feeling tense, then what does "can't stand" mean?	*Could it mean that I don't like feeling tense? Who does? Now, what can I do to address stressful issues?*
I must have immediate relief.	If you knew that this tension would lift in five minutes, would that be soon enough?	*Is it possible to view anxious discomfort as no more or less than a transient experience?*
I can't endure this any longer.	What makes you think that your ability to tolerate tension is limited?	*Endurance is limited by the limits I put on it.*

I won't be able to survive.	You've survived this tension before, so what makes you think that you won't live through it again?	*I definitely can survive what I don't like, and I can thrive by accepting the proposition that I can control my thoughts and actions to both cope and prosper.*

EXERCISE: QUESTION DRAMATIZED THINKING

Identify your distress beliefs, rationally question these beliefs, and provide answers in the space provided.

LFT Distress Beliefs	Your Questions	Your Answers
1.		
2.		
3.		
4.		
5.		
6.		

By questioning your thinking process whenever you have uncomfortable physical sensations and jump to negative conclusions about them, you can gain clarity and perspective on what is going on.

YOUR PROGRESS REPORT

Write down what you learned from this chapter and what actions you plan to take. Then record what resulted from taking these actions and what you've gained.

What are three key ideas that you took away from this chapter?

1.

2.

3.

What top three actions can you take to combat a specific anxiety or fear?

1.

2.

3.

What resulted when you took these actions?

1.

2.

3.

What did you gain from taking action? What would you do differently next time?

1.

2.

3.

CHAPTER 16

Vanquishing Panic

There is no mistaking panic. You gasp for breath. You tremble. You sweat, feel numb and unreal. You feel dizzy. You fear fainting, losing control, and going crazy. You think you are going to die, and this belief escalates the panic. You feel so frightened that you cry.

Although the physical symptoms of panic can seem sudden and uncontrollable, panic is a definable, explainable, and highly correctable condition. You can draw from a variety of CBT techniques to overcome panic, such as building self-efficacy beliefs for controlling panic (Gallagher et al. 2013) and using a combination of relaxation, breathing, and exposure techniques (Sánchez-Meca et al. 2010). Knowing how to defuse panicked thinking can quickly ease your panic. About two-thirds of those who combat panic make durable improvements (Gloster et al. 2013). You can do better!

PANIC FACTS

If you've gone through one or more panic episodes, you are not alone. Annually, between 3.5 percent and 10 percent of people between the ages of fifteen and sixty have serious persistent or isolated panic reactions (Barlow 1988; Katerndahl and Realini 1993; Kessler et al. 2012). As many as 40 percent of people over their lifetimes have some lower-grade symptoms or major panic symptoms (Bystritsky et al. 2010). If you have one of these subthreshold panic patterns, don't brush it aside. Minor panic is a risk factor for depression and other quality-of-life robbing conditions, such as substance abuse (Pané-Farré et al. 2013). Fortunately, CBT self-help manuals on panic can be helpful for those who suffer from panic (Lewis, Pearce, and Bisson 2012).

Panic Symptoms

The physical symptoms of panic can feel so severe that you may think you have a medical problem, but panic is usually psychologically addressable. Panic consists of not only physical symptoms but also cognitive triggers, emotional intolerance, and behavior avoidance issues. Muscular tension, chest pains, and gastrointestinal problems can be symptoms of anxiety as well as triggers for panic. Since these physical symptoms could reflect a medical problem, it would be wise to have a medical checkup, if you haven't already done so, to assure yourself that any persistent anxieties don't have a medication or disease connection. For example, a hyperactive thyroid condition can stimulate anxious feelings and thinking.

Panic Duration

Panic has a beginning, a middle, and an end. It doesn't go on forever. And, more often than not, it has a short duration. Panic can range from a short, unpleasant jolt of tension to a sudden and intense wave. Panic symptoms last usually between two and thirty minutes and closer to the two-minute mark. In rare instances, panicked feelings can last an hour or more. But even a few minutes of panic can seem like an eternity.

Panic typically follows a process that includes a sensation awareness phase, a cognitive trigger phase, a panic escalation phase, and a resolution phase. The good news is that you can attack negative panic thinking at any stage in this cycle, which will help you overcome it.

Panic Vs. Anxiety

When anxious, you are likely to experience muscle tension, headaches, or a nervous stomach. However, a sudden surge of tension, accompanied by dramatic physical symptoms, can feel so extreme that you experience a loss of control—as though you're free-falling and can't stop. Because of the dramatic nature of panic, you may feel anxious about panicking.

Two Forms of Panic

Panic comes in two major forms. *Uncued* panic appears unpredictable and seems to come out of the blue. *Cued panic* is where you panic only under specific situations, such as upon entering areas that you view as dangerous. It is also common that people link certain cues, such as lights, tone, and touch, to panic (Davis 1998).

Coping with Uncued Panic

Panic can come as a surprise without any obvious reason. However, there may be early and subtle panic signals. Behavioral therapy founder Joseph Wolpe (1967) found that 83 percent of the time, people who experience panic reactions have experienced significant tension the day before. He suggested a connection between a panic response and recently elevated stress hormones. Some studies have shown that higher than normal levels of epinephrine (a stress hormone) increase the risk for panic.

Even though uncued panic may come out of the blue, you can do something about it:

1. Think about your thinking and refuse to accept panicked thinking as fact. Thinking you are going crazy, for example, is a proposition, not a fact. Remind yourself of that.

2. Exercise emotional tolerance through an acceptant attitude. Acceptance can take this form: *If I panic, I panic. Tough. It's not the worst thing in the world.*

3. Engage behavioral measures to address panic, including breathing exercises, measuring the length of time that panic lasts, or making a mental note of the physical symptoms.

4. When you are in a calm state of mind, rehearse cognitive, emotional tolerance, and behavioral methods for dealing with panic, so you'll know what to do if panic returns.

You can use these same methods to cope with cued panic.

Coping with Cued Panic

With cued panic, you know what kicks off your fear, such as being in an elevator, a crowd, or an unfamiliar place. Looking down from a cliff can create a sense of dizziness that triggers panic. After being in a minor vehicle accident, you may panic when nearing the intersection where the accident occurred. Alternatively, you may panic in situations that remind you of a traumatic episode. You may have had a near-death experience. Cues from the event can include time of day, a special date, air temperature, a color, a smell, or a screeching sound. A client associated the sound of a helicopter with a near-death experience in a war zone and hid in panic whenever seeing or hearing a helicopter. Another associated hot weather with a terrifying death camp experience. He refused to leave his apartment in summer months when the temperature rose over eighty degrees.

If you are afraid that you'll lose your ability to think and act protectively when anxious, think again. Performance tests given during high fear arousal show that we can manage basic survival operations effectively. When you panic, blood flow actually increases to the right cerebral hemisphere, which enhances survival. At the same time, the blood supply to the left hemisphere is reduced. The resulting imbalance somewhat impedes your reasoning abilities, but you can still think clearly if you put your mind to the task.

Similarly, you may also fear any number of consequences—such as that you'll pass out, lose bowel control, or vomit—but these are rare events. You have about a 3 percent chance of any of these things happening while you are panicking (Green et al. 2007).

MANAGING PANIC

Accepting panic moderates the intensity and duration of panic. The trick is to get from panicking over panicking to acceptance and emotional tolerance of what you can honestly view as a highly unpleasant experience.

Coping with Interpretations

Panic doesn't happen in a vacuum. You'll likely have evaluative cognitions: you believe you'll look foolish; you think people will think you are crazy if you show signs of panicking. Such panic thoughts merit examination. For example, if you panic at restaurants and avoid eating out because you believe that you'll be seen and judged, here are some questions to ask yourself:

- Where is the evidence that all restaurant patrons will see you in the same way?

- Might some people view you with sympathy because they've experienced panic too?

- What is the likelihood that you won't be noticed?

Replace automatic negative cognitions with more positive realistic ideas about what might happen, and you will no longer avoid places that could conceivably cue panic.

Gaining Perspective

In situations where you experience a panic reaction for the first time, you can gain perspective by asking yourself if something has recently changed in your life situation. Stress accompanies life changes, including positive ones. Have you gone on a diet? Have you started taking a new medication? Have you had a recent trauma?

If you know the triggers, signs, and causes of panic, self-observation can replace a panicky reaction with a reflective response. Taking self-observant actions can be helpful: check your watch to see how long the panic reaction lasts. Make mental notes of the various aspects of the reaction: your thoughts, feelings, and behaviors.

Perhaps one of the best ways to understand and manage panic is to look at how a knowledgeable professional coped with this condition. Here's what Donna, a psychologist, did to address her panic.

• *Donna's Story*

Donna experienced a panic reaction following the recent deaths of three people she felt close to. When her panic started, she first felt sudden disturbing symptoms in her body. She described them as "waves of hot and cold spreading through my chest and down my arms and legs, tingling in my limbs, my heart beating fast, a feeling like I couldn't breathe, and sudden sweating. It hit me seemingly out of nowhere. Bam! My body was on red alert, and it felt awful."

She first thought she was having a heart attack: "I felt a new spurt of hot and cold pour through my skin. I took my pulse, and it was fast but steady. I have a home blood-pressure kit and took my blood pressure. It was a little high, but still normal. I did a symptom check. I found no pressure in my chest or any pain in chest or arm or jaw. The symptoms were on the surface, on my skin. I'd experienced such feelings before from adrenaline overload. I told myself I was likely having an anxiety attack, not a heart attack. If I couldn't abate the symptoms with a couple of minutes of REBT, I'd call an ambulance just in case it was a heart attack. But I was pretty certain it wasn't.

"My first step was to attend to my breathing. It was shallow and fast. I spent sixty seconds taking slow deep breaths. Since the symptoms lessened when I breathed correctly, I became more certain it was anxiety and not a heart attack. What had I been thinking? Then I tried to uncover the thoughts that had triggered the physical symptoms.

"The first thought that came to mind was that Tim was dead. Lou was dead. My brother had died two years ago. Everyone was dead, leaving behind relatives that I was supposed to support and help through their grief. That grief went on for months and months. It took so much out of me that I heard myself say, 'This was awful. I can't stand it anymore.'

"As I thought about the people around me, I thought, *I've had enough. They should not make any more demands on me. I should not have to deal with any of this awful stuff. They won't leave me alone to attend to my own life. All this death was awful. My husband has been having some health problems lately. He could be next. I can't stand the idea of being without him.*"

Donna recorded her thoughts as she sat by her computer. Then she started to reflect on her thinking. "The thought of my husband dying (when in fact he's no more close to dying than any of us) and me being a young widow was the tripping point for my anxiety attack. I realized that the thought had streaked through my mind like a meteor in daylight. I almost didn't register it consciously. But that was the final straw. It had triggered a fight-or-flight panic reaction in my body. My physical symptoms of anxiety were still intense but slightly less than a few minutes earlier.

"While still attending to my breathing, making sure I was not edging toward hyperventilation, I proceeded to rationally dispute each of my irrational beliefs. The 'I can't stand it' thoughts seem to be an especially strong trigger for me. My physical symptoms began to abate within seconds of identifying and then disputing this irrational self-talk.

"I continued to monitor my breathing and my thinking, disputing my awfulizing and catastrophic thinking and ending with a more rational view. True, things were bad. True, I had pressures on my time. But I could clearly see that taking a bad situation and making it worse, then getting myself anxious by catastrophizing about my husband's condition, had escalated my sense of terror. Fortunately, knowing what cognitions to look for, and knowing how to challenge them, came easily. I have practiced challenging them in calmer times, and that gives me a repertoire of rational self-talk to use in times of stress.

"After the worst symptoms had left me, I went to the kitchen and made myself a high protein drink and drank it slowly. Adrenal overload can cause severe fluctuations in blood sugar. This can cause further physical symptoms. A healthy drink with protein and complex carbs can prevent that. I took extra doses of B-complex vitamins. Maybe it was a placebo, but I believed that my fight-or-flight reaction used body stores of thiamine, pantothenic acid, and other B vitamins.

"I could smell myself. Anxiety sweat has a pungently bad odor. I took a shower, making an effort to enjoy the feeling of the hot water and the fragrance of my lavender soap. I told myself that even in the midst of loss and grief, I could still enjoy simple pleasures.

"While feeling the pleasantness of the hot shower, I continued disputing my awfulizing and catastrophizing. I reassured myself that although I did not like dealing with loss—and the grief that goes with it—I could stand it. By then, most of my symptoms were gone. I did continue to feel a little jangly inside, down in my abdomen. My chest felt fine. I told myself that the jangly feeling was the result of the sudden rush of adrenaline, a natural symptom. I could stand it. It was an inconvenience, not a catastrophe.

"I slept well that night. The next day, I had gastrointestinal distress, a normal symptom of the fight-or-flight response. Recognizing what was going on, I spared myself another bout of awfulizing and catastrophizing about my physical sensations. I also spent the day doing important tasks that I wanted to do and had been putting off due to my feeling that I must live up to my responsibilities to others. Instead, I engaged in behaviors to make my life better. I stacked another cord of firewood, took care of my garden, mowed the lawn, and went to the gym to work out—all things that I actually enjoy and which make my own life more manageable."

Getting a Grip on Panic

In dealing with her panic reaction, Donna took a series of productive steps:

1. She assessed her symptoms and came up with a plan for dealing with them.

2. She made a rational effort to distinguish anxiety from a more serious heart ailment.

3. She monitored her breathing, using a breathing technique to prevent an escalation of more unpleasant symptoms that can be brought on by shallow, fast breathing and/or hyperventilation.

4. She identified the irrational self-talk that had triggered the fight-or-flight response, and she replaced the irrational statements and beliefs with rational statements.

5. Because she had practiced recognizing and challenging anxiety-evoking beliefs in calm circumstances, she found it easier to automatically use Albert Ellis's ABCDE method (see chapter 11) in a stressful circumstance.

6. She engaged in self-care: eating, bathing, and comforting herself.

7. She accepted that her body would need several days to fully recover from the adrenaline overload.

8. When she suffered gastrointestinal distress the next day, she accepted it as a normal consequence of adrenaline overload. She did not make a federal case over a minor discomfort. Thus, she avoided rekindling her panic through anxiety sensitivity.

9. She actively engaged in behaviors that made her life more enjoyable and manageable.

10. She continued to monitor herself for shallow breathing and took a metacognitive approach to monitor her thinking for signs of irrational self-talk.

There are times when multiple pressures can get to even those who know better. But the real message from Donna's experience is that through knowledge and know-how, she brought this pattern of panic to a relatively quick end. She acted to prevent panic from coming back. You can employ the same techniques in overcoming panic reactions.

USING THE ABCDE METHOD FOR PANIC THINKING

The following ABCDE chart illustrates how to take catastrophic thoughts out of panic. By knowing how to do this, and practicing what you know, you can put yourself in charge of what you do when panicked.

ABCDE Method Applied to Panic Thinking

Activating event (experience): Experiencing physical sensations you associate with the onset of panic.

Reasonable beliefs about the event: "I've experienced these sensations before. They'll remain the same for a while, escalate, or diminish and disappear. The outcome is whatever the outcome is."

Emotional and behavioral consequences of the reasonable beliefs: A sense of emotional acceptance and tolerance about the experience. Possibly making adjustments in breathing or breathing into cupped hands to help recalibrate the CO_2 sensor in the brain.

Erroneous beliefs about the event: "Oh my god. It's happening again. I can't stand it. I'm about to die."

Emotional and behavioral consequences of the erroneous beliefs: A swelling of panic associated with the catastrophic fear of dying. Frenzied behavior. A 911 call.

Disputing erroneous beliefs:

1. What is the "it" that is happening again? Sample response: The likely "it" is both the fear of the feeling and the catastrophic anticipation that emotions and sensations of panic will be intolerable. Now, why can't you stand what you don't like? The answer is that you can stand what you don't like.

2. If panic is happening again, and you think you're going to die, then how is this view any different from before? Sample response: This experience is similar to panic you've experienced before, including the idea that you're about to die. You did not die that time. You just thought that you would. So, if you have a past history of surviving panic, why would you think that you wouldn't survive again? The answer is, you're highly likely to survive this experience. The threat is found in your catastrophic thoughts and not in reality. Focus on what you can control, which is refusing to cave into this alarmist thinking.

Effects of disputes: Decreasing the intensity of panic by changing the interpretation of the experience. Reducing the possibility of intensifying panic because you are catastrophizing about the symptoms and outcome. Following survival from panic, new conclusions are reasonable:

1. The fact that you can start to think differently when panic starts proves that you are not helpless.

2. Defusing catastrophic thinking decreases the intensity of panic and its durability.

3. The hormone storm passes without any durable ill effects; the same will happen if you panic again.

4. You still don't like feeling panic. Who would? But you now have more compelling evidence that the catastrophic prediction of dying is no more than a mental myth attached to panic sensations.

EXERCISE: ABCDE PRACTICE

Now it is your turn to use the ABCDE method to address panic thinking. Write down your adversity (or activating event), any beliefs (both reasonable and erroneous) that you have about the adversity, and the emotional and behavioral consequences of having these beliefs. Then dispute your erroneous beliefs, and see what happens. Finally, write down the effects of this process.

Your ABCDE Resolution

Activating event (experience):
Reasonable beliefs about the event:
Emotional and behavioral consequences of the reasonable beliefs:
Erroneous beliefs about the event:
Emotional and behavioral consequences of the erroneous beliefs:

Disputing erroneous beliefs:
Effects of disputes:

PANIC-CONTROL SIMULATION TECHNIQUES

Interoceptive exposure techniques are growing in popularity as a way to deal with each major physical part of panic. Using this exposure method, you learn that the different symptoms of panic are not dangerous, that they are tolerable, and that they may have a transdiagnostic effect across different negative emotional conditions (Boswell et al. 2013).

If you feel dizzy, you may believe that you are about to pass out. This belief can be especially troublesome when you are driving. But is it true? When panicked, dizziness doesn't predict fainting. Fainting occurs with a slow heartbeat. When you are panicked, your heart rate has increased. Panic normally protects you against fainting.

Dizziness is easily simulated. Here is a common technique. Spin yourself in a chair enough times to show yourself that however dizzy you get, you won't faint. You may even conclude that fainting is preferable to dizziness.

The quickened heartbeat of panic is only dramatic when compared to a resting heart rate. If you were panicked and took your pulse rate, you would probably discover that it's about what you'd expect if you were exercising. The sudden change is the alarming factor (primal fears typically start with a sudden and unexpected threat event).

A quickened heartbeat is easy to simulate. Do moderate exercise to bring your heart rate to between 120 and 140 beats per minute. This is a common panic-level heart rate, and well below a dangerous tachycardia of around 200 beats per minute.

Hyperventilation is attempting to breathe in air beyond a metabolic need, and it commonly occurs in panic. Panicking over your breathing difficulties can add to panic.

Hyperventilating also is easily simulated. For example, breathing through a straw with your nose pinched shut can simulate a panic symptom of gasping for air. Through this process, you can show yourself that when you hyperventilate, nothing happens. You'll feel forced to return to normal breathing within a short time.

In using simulation techniques to intentionally experience aspects of a panic reaction, you can show yourself that the symptoms of panic are not overwhelming. This knowledge can help quell panicked thinking about dizziness, heart rate, and breathing.

BREAKING THE AGORAPHOBIA-PANIC CONNECTION

About one-third of those who suffer from panic suffer from agoraphobia, which largely boils down to a fear of panic and avoidance of situations that are associated with panic.

The physical, cognitive, emotional, and behavioral facets of panic can be so dramatic that you avoid situations that you associate with panic. You'll avoid restaurants, riding in buses, flying in planes, shopping at the mall—anywhere that you fear you'll be in danger, trapped, and helpless if you panic. You may remain housebound out of fear that you may panic wherever you go; you may venture out only if someone goes with you to support you.

The situations that you fear aren't dangerous; you probably already know that. You're afraid of yourself—panicking and losing control. You are afraid of how you'll look to others. You worry, *What if I fell to pieces while waiting in line?*

By avoiding or escaping from panic situations and consequently feeling a sense of relief, you are reinforcing avoidance. Similarly, if you have panic reactions, you may create crutches for yourself. For example, you might distract yourself with loud music piped through earphones. You might bring an antidepressant pill with you if you know you have little choice but to venture into an unsafe area. If these distractions ease your tension and reinforce their use, sooner or later you are likely to discover that there is an unpleasant downside. You are priming yourself to avoid or escape panic and reinforcing the wrong behavior.

A big part of the solution is to learn to live through panic without avoiding it. If you teach yourself how not to fear panic, you are unlikely to panic over the possibility of panicking.

EXERCISE: TURNING DISTRACTIONS INTO PRODUCTIVE ACTIONS

Next time you feel panic coming on, follow these three steps to turn distractions into productive actions.

1. Label catastrophic thoughts, such as *I will collapse* or *I will die*, as *panic thinking*. Remind yourself that these thoughts will eventually fade like a whistle in a canyon.

2. Wait out the physical symptoms and sensations of panic until the sensations subside. This can be tough to do. However, trying to escape the feelings reinforces escape. You are going through an anxiety cycle. You might as well accept it.

3. Take behavioral actions, such as taking your pulse rate and timing how long the panic takes to subside. However, you use this distraction to gather information—not as an escape.

You may discover that what you have been dramatizing makes an unpleasant situation worse. When your dramatize a situation, it is not as bad as you think.

Top Tip: A Paradoxical Way to Control Panic

Dr. Rick Paar is a professor of psychology at Springfield College. He has a creative flair, which he put to good use when he once suffered excruciating panic. Fortunately, with his legacy and personal knowledge, he went to work on himself right away. Rick shares what he did to control his panic:

"I have never been a fan of flying. I do it, but I don't like it. About ten years ago, three of my graduate students and I had some papers accepted at the International Congress on Psychotherapy in Italy, and since there was no way I could drive to Europe, flying from Boston to Rome was the only option.

"The international terminal at Logan Airport is gigantic, easily the size of four or five football fields, so I can't say that I felt a sense of claustrophobia in the place, but I surely felt sweaty and uncomfortable as I went through customs and couldn't turn around and go home. It was a little later that I began to feel a small wave of panic rise from my belly and, with it, a voice that whispered in my head, *What if you freak out? You can't do that. You must not do that.* And, of course, the more I said that, the more anxious I became. I thought of how lame I would look in front of my students and how stupidly ironic it was that we were going to a conference to talk about psychotherapy.

"I tried walking from one end of the terminal to the other. I tried sitting and breathing. I tried thinking of other things. And nothing worked. All I got was more and more anxious. Finally, I decided to make myself have the biggest damned panic attack anyone has ever seen.

"*Go on, do it. Do it!* And of course I couldn't. So then I said, *Okay, in seventeen minutes try it again*, which nicely gave me seventeen minutes of relief. And when seventeen minutes were gone, I tried to have the biggest damned panic attack one more time, and again I couldn't. So, I picked another odd number of minutes, thirteen or nineteen or something, and again I had relief. I did this a few more times until it felt silly. A while later, we boarded the plane which, of course, sat on the tarmac for three and a half hours before we took off. I stretched out and read a book."

YOUR PROGRESS REPORT

Write down what you learned from this chapter and what actions you plan to take. Then record what resulted from taking these actions and what you've gained.

What are three key ideas that you took away from this chapter?

1.

2.

3.

What top three actions can you take to combat a specific anxiety or fear?

1.

2.

3.

What resulted when you took these actions?

1.

2.

3.

What did you gain from taking action? What would you do differently next time?

1.

2.

3.

CHAPTER 17

Combatting Simple Phobias and Fears

Karen has a morbid fear of germs and goes to extremes to avoid contamination. Abby panics about snakes and refuses to go outside when there is any possibility of encountering one. Lloyd is afraid of dogs. When his best friend got a pet dog, Lloyd refused to go anywhere near it. What do Karen, Abby, and Lloyd have in common? They all have a serious specific phobia, or a persistent fear of an animal, situation, object, or other event that they go out of their way to avoid.

Phobias are common. In any one year, 8.7 percent of the US population will have a serious phobic reaction to one thing or another. The lifetime prevalence estimate is 12.1 percent (Kessler et al. 2005). Phobias include fears of natural disasters, animals, insects, injections and blood, flying, public speaking, and social events, such as attending parties, family gatherings, or weddings.

Some phobias are more of a quirk than a handicap. For example, you may have a phobia of the number thirteen (triskaidekaphobia). Whatever the reason, you may avoid living on the thirteenth floor of a building, or flinch a bit on Friday the thirteenth, but otherwise this fear is no big deal to you. Even the great Babylonian King Hammurabi avoided labeling his thirteenth law with the number thirteen. He skipped over it, going from twelve to fourteen. However, if you have a debilitating fear of the number thirteen, it's not silly. Any phobia that interferes with the quality of your life merits attention.

You can sometimes overcome a debilitating phobia in a surprisingly short time and get a transdiagnostic bonus. By acting to overcome your phobias and fears, you can buffer yourself against other anxieties (Indovina et al. 2011).

PUTTING YOURSELF IN CONTACT WITH WHAT YOU FEAR

What you need to do to overcome your phobia is relatively simple but not necessarily easy. That is because overcoming a phobia is more of a process than a single event, especially if you have a network of complications interconnecting with your phobia. If you don't know whether what you have is a fear or a phobia, it may not matter. Both fears and phobias tend to follow similar neurological paths (Schweckendiek et al. 2011). The same CBT methods that are effective for overcoming fears are effective for overcoming phobias.

Exposure-based CBT is the gold standard for addressing phobias and fears. Here are some basic steps in this process:

1. Educate yourself. Learn about common causes for phobias and evidence-based solutions.

2. Agree with yourself that you'll learn to tolerate tension until you no longer fear the feeling of fear that you associate with your parasitic fear situation.

3. Put yourself in proximity to what you fear, in tolerable chunks, one step at a time.

4. You will have a natural impulse to avoid what you fear. This avoidance rarely does more than reinforce itself and perpetuate the fear. Resist it!

5. Persist until you have control over yourself in the proximity of what you fear.

These basic steps will help you overcome any phobia. This chapter elaborates on how to use them in different ways and in different situations.

Addressing a Germ Phobia

It's good to be health conscious and to take prudent steps to prevent health problems. However, a good thing can be taken to an unhealthy extreme. If you have a germ phobia, you have an unhealthy concern with protecting yourself from practically everything that could carry germs. Germ phobias range from mild and somewhat troublesome to the extreme displayed by the billionaire Howard Hughes, who confined himself to small sterile quarters to avoid germs and contamination.

Even when you know you have a germ phobia, you rarely can simply order it out of existence. You'll have to work your way out.

• Karen's Story

Karen had a morbid fear of germs. This ordinarily friendly social scientist believed that unless she was extraordinarily cautious, she would contract a deadly disease and possibly die. As a result, she panicked whenever she believed that she'd been exposed to germs.

Her presenting problem was not only her fear of germs. Her friendships were strained, and she wanted to know how to communicate better. It was clear, however, that her refusal to join her friends at restaurants and gatherings because she was afraid of germs had alienated the people whom she loved best. Her germ phobia was interfering with her relationships and her peace of mind.

When gently approached about this matter, Karen snapped, "Germs Kill!" When it became plain enough to Karen that she going nowhere by denying her problem, she put on her scientist's hat and experimented her way out of her problem.

She worked—uncomfortably at first—at taking away one safety behavior a week. For example, to protect herself from germs, she had been wearing Teflon gloves everywhere she went. As a condition for removing the gloves, she first used an antibiotic hand cleaner every hour. Then she scaled this back until she washed her hands before and at other appropriate times. She substituted a short-sleeved blouse during summertime for the heavy sweaters she'd been wearing. She had originally thought that long sleeves protected her from germs.

By making problem-related behavioral changes and becoming comfortable with these changes, Karen shed her fear of dying from germs. She rebuilt her friendships. This process took about six months.

For Karen, the process of overcoming her phobia involved a series of turning points. Her first turning point was seeing the contradiction between her scientific training and her unscientific acceptance of the belief that she was in imminent danger of being killed by germs. Her second turning point was acceptance of her panic feelings. Her third turning point came when she saw that she was not a slave to her fear and could overcome it if she tried.

Addressing a Snake Phobia

What do you do to quell a phobia of snakes or other animals, bugs, open spaces, or entrapment? How can you normalize your life in this area? Controlled exposure experiences may be the most effective thing that you can do to overcome such fears. This means to get in proximity to situations where you know—or suspect—that you are exaggerating a danger.

• Abby's Story

Abby was housebound because of her fear of snakes. She wouldn't go to her daughter's school events. She arranged to have teacher conferences on her computer through FaceTime. Her therapy sessions were by telephone. Her reason for these restrictions was that she might be attacked and bitten by a poisonous snake. Her daughter's excuse for her, "that's just Mom being Mom," had an unsettling effect on her. She wanted relief from this burden. The time had come to take action.

Abby decided to use exposure to defuse her snake phobia. She decided to take a graduated approach. She liked the idea of training her primitive brain to stop overreacting to her images of snakes.

Her goal was to feel free to leave her home without dreading snakes. She believed that her phobia of snakes was the cause of her panic. Arguably, it was her fear of losing control and panicking that was the primary issue, but her exposure program would help her overcome this fear as well. Specifically, Abby believed that if she could walk daily through a local park, she could go just about anywhere, so walking through a local park was her goal.

Abby's first step was looking at pictures of nonpoisonous snakes at a comfortable distance in the confines of her home. She used the family room because she found that room relaxing and pleasant. She would move a foot at a time, from one end of the room to the other, where her daughter had put a snake picture. She proceeded until she could hold the snake picture and look at the snake up close.

She went to a reptile exhibit at a museum to observed stuffed snakes behind a glass exhibit. She planned to use the same procedure as she did with the picture. However, she had to get to the museum. During the trip, she suffered high anxiety as her husband drove her. Her two daughters, who were accompanying her, offered encouragement. By design, her husband dropped her and the two girls at the stairs in front of the museum entrance. She briskly walked through the door and to the exhibit cases. She put herself within three feet of the snake exhibit case. She looked at all the snakes, including the poisonous variety. By the time her husband joined her, she was giddy. Approaching the snake exhibit was manageable.

Next, Abby drove with her family to observe snakes in the local zoo reptile exhibit. The live snakes were housed in glass cases. As before, she briskly moved closer to the case. She wanted to finish the exercise quickly. She found she was interested in the colors of the snakes and reported learning a lot from what was written about them. She struck up a conversation with a fellow visitor who had a few pet snakes. She found her fears manageable and also found that they decreased the longer she stayed at the zoo. When she felt relaxed, she left.

Her next step was to wear tall leather boots and walk around her lawn. She did this with her family. She felt safe from a snake with the boots protecting her legs. She felt she could handle the tension, so she walked around her block by herself.

Next, she wore ankle-high boots as she walked around her lawn and then around the block. Once she felt relaxed with this process, she repeated the exercise wearing sneakers.

Finally, on her own, she walked through the park, wearing boots. Thereafter, she walked in sneakers with her family around the park.

How long does exposure take to work? For Karen, it took six months. For Abby, it was over and done in a few days. Everyone is different. The answer to how long it takes to stop feeling phobic is that it takes as long as it takes.

A CLASSIC APPROACH TO OVERCOMING PHOBIAS

The classic approach for overcoming a phobia or fear has six steps: start with a goal, set up a hierarchy, practice relaxation, create coping statements, imagine exposure steps, and take exposure steps.

Start with a Goal

Your goal should be meaningful, reasonable, measurable, and accomplishable. For example, if you were Lloyd, with a dog phobia, what would you want to accomplish? Would it be to own a big aggressive dog? Would you want to be able to walk past a large dog with no more than normal wariness? Would you want to be able to pet a large friendly dog? Would you want to feel at ease around companion dogs that seem to be friendly? Before we get to Lloyd's case, let's look at typical steps for setting up a program to address a phobia. I'll use a dog phobia as an example.

Set Up a Hierarchy

Identify mild, moderate, and severe fear situations and arrange them from least to most scary. If you were afraid of dogs, the least scary image might be a small dog who acts friendly; you might imagine a twinge of anxiety if you saw this dog at the end of your driveway lying down and being held on a leash by its owner. This image will be the first step on your hierarchy. Create a second item for your list. This might be the same dog, same situation, except this time the dog is sitting. This image should be slightly more tension producing than the first one. The final step on your hierarchy may be you holding the small dog. In setting up your hierarchy, it's good to keep the degree of tension about equal between steps.

Practice a Relaxation Technique

Use a relaxation technique to achieve a calm state. You may want to refer to a relaxation technique from chapter 9 or another source. Practice relaxing until you can produce the desired effect.

Create Coping Statements for Each Step

Come up with coping statements that will work for each step of exposure. A self-efficacy belief such as "I can organize and regulate my actions to achieve my goal" may do. The idea is to identify coping statements that will help you to maintain a coping perspective during exposure.

Imagine Exposure

In a relaxed state of mind and in a relaxed position, imagine the first step on your hierarchy. Think of your coping statement. Repeat this relax–image–coping statement process until you feel comfortable with the image. Then move on in your mind to the next step on your hierarchy.

How often should you practice this visualizing technique? Your best gauge is what you can comfortably do each day. When you are comfortable with the top image on your hierarchy, you can move on to live exposure.

Take Live Exposure Steps

Start with the first step. Then move on to the next and so on until you have taken all the steps on your hierarchy and overcome your phobia. You might arrange doing this with someone you trust.

Top Tip: Overcome Your Phobia with the Help of a Friend

Few go through life without having a few fears and phobias. Dr. Howard Kassinove, Hofstra University professor of psychology and coauthor of *Anger Management for Everyone: Seven Proven Ways to Control Anger and Live a Happier Life*, acquired a phobia that restricted his enjoyment of one of his favorite activities. He tells what he did to overcome his phobia and how you can do the same:

"In psychotherapy, we talk about the importance of the therapeutic alliance. By that, we mean that progress is often based on trust and respect for the therapist. We have to believe that person is working on our behalf, to help. That concept has been central in helping me overcome some of my own anxieties.

"Many years ago, I developed a fear of heights after trying unsuccessfully to learn how to become a pilot. I had a few terrifying close calls. The fear generalized to ski lifts, and I became "unable" to go on any lifts that left the ground. Although I avoided a favorite pastime, skiing, I wanted to return to it.

"I put myself on a program of desensitization. I went to various ski areas where the lifts took me progressively higher, culminating in very high lifts in the Colorado mountains. The secret to success for me was that I always went with a friend that I respected and trusted. I felt safe and secure and was willing to approach the previously avoided feared situation. It worked, and after a while, I could go on the lifts by myself.

"Recently, I made a trip to Hong Kong and was required to take a very high and very long gondola ride to the top of a mountain. I accomplished the task with ease.

"I recommend working on your phobia with someone you trust, respect, and even admire. It can go a long way."

• *Lloyd's Story*

Lloyd's neighbor had a small friendly dog. She knew Lloyd was afraid of dogs because Lloyd would duck into his house whenever she went outside with the dog. Otherwise, Lloyd and his neighbor enjoyed a good relationship. He sometimes joked with her that he'd someday pet her dog. She invited him—on numerous occasions—to approach the dog.

When Lloyd decided he wanted to overcome his fear of dogs, he explained to his neighbor what he was trying to accomplish. His goal was to be able to pet a small friendly dog. His neighbor was delighted to help. The following day, he gave her a copy of the exposure steps to his hierarchy, explaining that he would have to prepare himself mentally before taking each step.

His plan was to take eight minutes for each exposure step. He would use two minutes to conjure the image of the first exposure step while pairing it with deep breathing. At the end of that time, he would repeat the coping statement three times in his mind. Then he would take the first step for five minutes of exposure. After that he would allow a minute to wind down. If he felt okay with this step, he'd take the next step, and so on. If not, he'd repeat the step.

Lloyd succeeded in overcoming his dog phobia from small dogs. Despite this initial success, Lloyd wasn't done with his program. He visited and observed several dog obedience classes and attended dog shows. He's still vigilant when it comes to meeting a strange dog that growls, as he should be. Otherwise, he's comfortable around companion dogs of any size.

OVERCOMING YOUR PHOBIA

It's time to take steps to overcome your phobia. First set your goal and then create an exposure hierarchy. You can use Lloyd's hierarchy as a model; it includes four classic phases: relaxation technique, imagery, coping statement, and exposure:

Lloyd's Exposure Hierarchy

Relaxation Technique	Imagery	Coping Statement	Exposure
1. Deep breathing	Small, friendly neighborhood dog on leash	"I know this dog. He has never hurt anyone before."	Your neighbor brings her dog to the end of your driveway.
2. Deep breathing	Same small, friendly neighborhood dog on leash nearby	"This dog is friendly and doesn't bite."	Your neighbor brings her dog to within one foot of you at your house.
3. Deep breathing	Same small, friendly dog at your house off leash	"This dog is friendly and doesn't bite."	Your neighbor walks her dog to your house and takes him off the leash for one minute.
4. Deep breathing	Same small, friendly dog; you take it for a walk around your house, on the leash.	"This dog is friendly and doesn't bite."	You take the dog for a walk of five minutes around your house several times until you feel relaxed.
5. Deep breathing	Take a walk around your neighborhood with a friend. Keep walking until you see at least one dog.	"These dogs are on leashes or fenced in and can't hurt me."	Walk around the neighborhood with a friend for at least a half hour.
6. Deep breathing	Repeat step 5 by yourself.	"I've already done this easily with my friend. I can do it on my own."	Walk around your neighborhood by yourself for at least a half hour or until you see several dogs and still feel relaxed.

EXERCISE: SETTING UP YOUR EXPOSURE HIERARCHY

Apply a hierarchical approach to your phobia. List your least scary situation as your first step, a situation that is slightly scarier as the next step, and so on until you describe your exposure goal. Include a relaxation technique, imagery, and a coping statement for each exposure step. Then proceed through the steps until you have sufficiently reduced or overcome your phobia.

Relaxation Technique	Imagery	Coping Statement	Exposure
1.			
2.			
3.			
4.			
5.			
6.			
7.			

YOUR PROGRESS REPORT

Write down what you learned from this chapter and what actions you plan to take. Then record what resulted from taking these actions and what you've gained.

What are three key ideas that you took away from this chapter?

1.

2.

3.

What top three actions can you take to combat a specific anxiety or fear?

1.

2.

3.

What resulted when you took these actions?

1.

2.

3.

What did you gain from taking action? What would you do differently next time?

1.

2.

3.

CHAPTER 18

A Multimodal Attack on Anxiety and Fear

Rutgers University professor emeritus Arnold Lazarus pioneered a multimodal therapy approach to help people combat anxiety and other undesirable conditions. Lazarus uses the acronym BASIC ID to describe seven *modalities*, or aspects of a problem condition, for understanding and overcoming anxiety: behavior, affect, sensation, imagery, cognitions, interpersonal, and drugs/biology (Lazarus 1992).

This chapter first introduces the BASIC-ID approach and then shows how to apply it to in a situation where your anxiety signals that you need to make some changes.

PRESCRIPTIONS FOR CHANGE

The BASIC-ID approach allows you to address each modality with a prescription for change:

1. *Behavior* refers to what you want to stop doing, such as retreating from your fears, or what you want to start doing, such as meeting worthy challenges.

2. *Affect* refers to your emotions. You may want to decrease negative affects, such as anxiety or harmful anger. You may want to increase moments of satisfaction and happiness.

3. *Sensations* refer to what you see and hear. But they also refer to anxiety-related sensations, including headaches, lower back pain, and gastrointestinal distress.

4. *Imagery* refers to pictures you have in your mind, such as a caricature of yourself, a fantasy, or a self-image.

5. *Cognitions* include your beliefs, attitudes, opinions, values, and philosophy.

6. *Interpersonal* refers to relationships that you have with others.

7. *Drugs/biology* includes medications you are on, substances you may abuse, health concerns, or biological tendencies toward anxiety or depression. This modality also includes brain issues.

From person to person, these modalities can vary in their order of importance. For example, you may be especially sensitive to your sensations. If you have a surprising increase in your heart rate, this sensation can trigger a panic cognition: *I'm having a heart attack, and I'm going to die.* You can then have an image of yourself in an ambulance heading to the hospital. This image can add to the increased heart rate and breathing problems. The above combination would be an S-C-I-D (sensation, cognition, imagery, and drugs/biology) pattern. Whatever your anxiety pattern, the BASIC-ID is a framework to break it down by priority issue and address it.

ANXIETY AS A HELPFUL SIGNAL FOR CHANGE

Anxiety can sometimes be a helpful signal for change. When you have natural anxiety, it's important to take your feelings of unease as warnings and respond in a timely way. However, sometimes you may have a hard time distinguishing between natural anxiety and unhealthy anxiety patterns. This was true for a client named Diana.

• *Diana's Story*

Diana was a twenty-three-year-old single woman who complained of severe anxiety and panic. Dwelling on her worries, she often had trouble falling asleep. She lacked exercise and often found herself gasping for air when climbing stairs. Otherwise, she was in good health. She did not use drugs or alcohol to deal with her tensions. She was not on any medications. Her weight was normal. Her appearance was attractive, her demeanor warm and engaging.

Diana said her anxieties controlled her life. She frequently panicked. She feared losing control and going crazy. She dreaded such feelings and said she would do practically anything to make them go away. She reported that often her muscles felt tense and her stomach was tied in knots. She couldn't think straight. She had difficulty concentrating. She was forgetful. She feared doing the wrong thing and being criticized. She was afraid to offend anyone. She felt insecure and riddled with self-doubts. She described herself as a fearful person. Where did her anxieties start? Diana described her early childhood as filled with pleasant memories and largely anxiety-free. Her description of that period seemed reasonable.

When she was a young adolescent, her anxiety had escalated. She was hypersensitive about making mistakes, looking like a fool, and getting rejected. During this period, she had an insight. She thought that to be liked, she would need to cater to other people's interests. Perhaps then they wouldn't pick up on her imperfections. Perhaps she could avoid conflict.

After a brief relationship and on her twenty-third birthday, she became engaged to Jack. Around that time, her anxieties jumped through the roof. Diana said that prior to the engagement, Jack seemed solicitous and attentive, and maybe a little jealous, at times, but in a charming way. Sure, he drank a tad too much. He said he needed to knock down a few cool ones to relax. She told herself, *That's a guy thing.*

Once she announced a wedding date, Diana moved into Jack's apartment. At that point, his jealousy increased. He demanded that she tell him where she was going and keep in constant touch with him by cell phone. He literally followed her around the apartment. Jack's drinking also increased. After three months of living with Jack, Diana felt confused about her feelings toward him.

Separating Unhealthy Anxieties from Natural Anxieties

Sometimes it can be difficult to separate unhealthy anxieties from natural ones, especially if you have had anxiety problems for a long time. For example, Diana had already experienced unhealthy anxiety before she met Jack, but her symptoms increased after she met him.

At first, Diana denied there was any connection between the rise in her anxiety and her relationship with Jack. She attributed it to prenuptial tension. Yet she broke into a sweat when she talked about her fiancé's tracking her every move and his uncontrolled drinking.

Initially, she doubted and blamed herself for what had happened. She recalled that at the beginning of their relationship, Jack was pleasant and attentive, but over time, his behavior had changed. It had to be her fault, she thought. He now knew the real Diana. Knowing her was driving him to drink. However, if drinking was a "guy thing," then how was she driving him to drink?

After taking a self-observant view, Diana realized that she was in an unhealthy relationship. She recalled pleading with him to trust her, but that plea got her nowhere. Jack had continued to hound her every move. She couldn't reason with him about his drinking. He told her to stop complaining. He had it under control.

Diana soon figured out that Jack had serious problems that would not be fixed by pleasing him or trying to work things out with him. Still, her relationship with Jack represented the lesser of two evils. She feared that no one else would marry her. She would end up alone. She had a gruesome image of her future. She saw herself as a wrinkled spinster surrounded by pet cats.

Shifting Perspective

When there is more than one way to view a situation, an *incongruity intervention* can help cause a shift in thinking, as you contrast an anxiety perspective with a realistic alternative view.

For example, Diana feared that others would see her as a failure if she broke off her engagement. She understood that she would never be happy with Jack, but she felt socially embarrassed at the thought of cancelling the wedding. She had already announced to her family and friends that Jack was a wonderful man and that she was very lucky to have found him. Would she sound like a hypocrite if she cancelled the wedding? She imagined her friends and family rolling their eyes in disapproval.

Shifting perspective, Diana recognized that if her best friend left an unhealthy relationship, she'd see this as a mark of courage. If she could accept that her friend could exit an unhealthy relationship without being a hypocrite and a failure, then why would she see herself as a hypocrite and a failure? As she faced this cognitive incongruity, she concluded that the fear that everyone would see her as a failure was a figment of her imagination.

Diana also did a reality check. She asked her mother and two close friends to give her their honest opinion of Jack. Her mother was blunt. Jack's drinking pattern was obvious and serious. She worried about Diana's future with Jack. She had planned to tell her daughter to delay the wedding and preferably break off the engagement. Both of Diana's friends said she should drop Jack. That ended her fear of public embarrassment about cancelling the wedding.

Diana considered her dating history before Jack entered her life. She was physically attractive. She had an engaging personality. She had dated often. Now she faced another incongruity. How could she be doomed to a life of spinsterhood when she'd previously had many suitors? Diana quickly saw that the spinster image didn't jibe with experience.

Taking Action

Even when you know what is best for you, it may take a while before you act on that knowledge. For example, Diana had accepted that she could never be happy with Jack, but she waded through several weeks of viewing herself as a bad person if she were to hurt Jack's feelings. She feared that Jack would get angry with her, resent her, and reject her if she called off the wedding. She imagined him towering over her shouting, "How could you do this to us? You promised to marry me." As a result, she continued to work on the relationship, hoping she could get through to Jack about her wishes to be an independent partner, but he didn't listen.

Diana faced another incongruous situation: if she couldn't get through to Jack, and he had already rejected her ideas and wishes for an equal partnership, what she feared most had already been realized. She decided that she could not control Jack's thoughts about her. She could probably never please Jack, however hard she tried, and especially when he prioritized drinking over their relationship.

Through exploring her fear of rejection, Diana came to realize that she probably had a strong fear of confrontation. Her strategy had been to duck conflict through appeasement, but that was about to change. At a crowded restaurant, Diana told Jack that the wedding was off. She picked a public setting because she knew that Jack would not make a scene. However, Jack persuaded her to give him a second chance. She suggested that he seek counseling, and he agreed.

For a short while, Jack was on his best behavior. He cut down on his drinking. He was less inquisitive about her whereabouts. Within three weeks, however, he had dropped counseling and resumed his old patterns. Diana's anxiety escalated, but this time she recognized that her anxiety was about her future with Jack.

Once she cleared through her mental anxiety clutter, Diana was better able to trust her real feelings. She accepted that her anxiety was a signal that the relationship was not right for her. She made the final break, and she had fewer anxieties to contend with.

BREAKING DOWN ANXIETY INTO MODALITIES

Taking a BASIC-ID approach can help you break down a complex anxiety problem and address both unhealthy and natural anxieties. This chart shows how Diana used a BASIC-ID approach to customize her change program. Note that Diana's BASIC-ID modality plan starts with cognition, since this modality was most important to her. However, some modalities overlap: her imagery included thoughts and perspectives that, when changed, neutralized a negative self-image.

Diana's BASIC-ID Modality Program

Modality	Problem Assessment	Prescription
Cognitions	1. *I can avoid conflict and rejection by pleasing others.* 2. *Cancelling the wedding will make me a failure in the eyes of others.*	1. Incongruity intervention: if you can accept that others won't be 100 percent pleasing, then why can't you accept that different people can have different interests in specific topics, and that's a normal part of life? A sample answer: unless you grew up in a fanatical cult, differences in opinions, perceptions, and perspective are normal. 2. If your best friend ended an unhealthy relationship, you would see it as a brave thing to do. Seek opinions from others as a reality check.

Imagery	1. Image of self as wrinkled spinster 2. Self-image of a fearful person	1. Picture yourself as a person succeeding and coping effectively. Picture yourself as a heroine. Decide what the heroine would do under trying circumstances, and play out the role. 2. Write out a script of what you tell yourself when you feel anxious. Carry on a dialogue in your mind between educated reason and anxiety talk.
Interpersonal	Avoiding conflicts and rejection at all cost	Risk standing up for your rights. Risk expressing your views and opinions.
Behavior	Making up excuses for others' poor behavior	1. Hold people accountable for destructive behaviors. 2. Avoid taking the blame for others' problem habits. 3. When appropriate, speak up for your rights.
Sensations	Tension, stiff muscles	Get massage. Do stretch exercises. Listen to relaxing music. Take a warm bath. Tighten and relax all major muscle groups in sequence.
Affect	1. Anxiety 2. Natural anxieties	1. Punch holes in such beliefs as *I'll be hated if I don't please others.* Use incongruity intervention: "If my mother and best friends did something I didn't like, would I hate them forever? If not, then why conclude that I have to be 100 percent perfect and curry 100 percent favor or lose all of my primary relationships? Who's to say that if I'm not perfect, I can't enjoy my primary relationships?" 2. Heed natural anxieties as warnings and respond in a timely and appropriate way. Rather than hide and procrastinate, take steps to cope!

| Drugs/biology | 1. Lack of exercise

2. Poor sleep patterns | 1. Engage in moderate exercise program: bicycle to work each day. Do an aerobic program at health spa.

2. Two hours before going to bed, take a warm bath. List the evidence to support worry thinking and then note contradictory facts, information, or beliefs. Use this information to counter worry thinking if it starts around bedtime. |

EXERCISE: CREATING YOUR BASIC-ID BLUEPRINT FOR CHANGE

To start your BASIC-ID program, write down a prime anxiety or fear. Then answer the questions to examine each modality of your problem.

Target anxiety or fear: _____.

Behavior: What are you doing to impede your own health and happiness? Write it down. What you would like to start doing? For example, would you like to act more assertively?

Affect: What negative emotions impact your psychic life? What generates these negative affects? Is it cognitions, imagery, interpersonal conflicts, or what? How do you act when you feel anxious?

Sensation: What sensations do you associate with your anxieties and fears? For example, do you tend to panic when you feel irregularities in your heartbeat?

Imagery: How do you picture yourself when you are in a state of distress? Do you have a negative self-image?

Cognition: What are your main anxiety or fear beliefs? For example, do you believe your problems will never end?

Interpersonal: How do you manage relationships? Do you place demands on others? Do you avoid social contacts?

Drugs/biology: What do you do to quell your tension? Do you smoke or drink when tense? Do you take a walk to calm down?

Now using the BASIC-ID framework, organize your information in the middle column under "problem assessment" in this worksheet. Since the same problems can appear in more than one modality, you'll have to make judgment calls about what information goes where. The important thing is to put key components of your anxiety or fear into an organized framework. Next, devise and record prescriptive plans for each modality problem, using techniques from this book or of your own invention.

Your BASIC-ID Program

Modality	Problem Assessment	Prescription
Behavior		
Affect		
Sensations		
Imagery		
Cognitions		
Interpersonal		
Drugs/biology		

If you wish, number the modalities in their order of importance to you, so you can prioritize what to address first, second, and so on. Based on your readiness level, execute your program, step by step.

Top Tip: Accelerate Your Path to Mastery

Multimodal therapist Dr. Jeffrey A. Rudolph shares this tip that he uses with his clients:

"Anxiety is like a warning light on your car's instrument panel. What does your anxiety signal tell you about what's happening when you feel anxious? The event may be clear in your mind. You have an overdue mortgage bill and can't make the payment. You have a sudden, unexplained abdominal pain. But other than a feeling of dread, you may not be aware of other key components of your anxiety.

"Start with a quick checkup. What's going on in your behavior, affect-emotion, sensation, imagery, cognition-thinking, interpersonal-social, and drugs-biological-health modalities? Next, for each relevant modality, create a practical and BASIC-ID problem-solving approach that is tailored to your personality and to the unique elements of the situation that you find challenging.

"Know your problem-solving assets. The multimodal psychotherapy approach is a personal health and resource-based approach that emphasizes what is right about you and what you can do to help yourself. For example, how many times have you faced a fearful situation where you first doubted yourself, but you persisted and overcame a painful adversity? Compile a ledger of past events where you faced a challenging problem—one that elicited anxiety—and where you overcame your anxieties and fears. Renew this ledger whenever you need to remind yourself that you have met anxiety before, overcome obstacles, and moved on feeling stronger.

"Use anxiety as a coping-skill opportunity to build competence and confidence. Here's a four-step process that my clients have found helpful:

1. Respect and honor your basic needs. The best way to fight anxiety is to seek out what gives you emotional fulfillment. You are most anxiety prone when your helpless beliefs disconnect you from your beliefs in your ability to execute your positive capabilities. Remember: stop protecting and start expressing.

2. Reflect by taking a step back to regain your perspective and to reconnect to your ledger of affirmative experiences where your persistence paid. Tune into your natural strengths.

3. Select the most powerful tools particularly molded to your needs. Plan your approach and remember your options.

4. Project positive imagery before confronting a challenging situation. By picturing yourself as capably managing the conditions of your anxieties, and putting to practice what is within your ability to do, with a bit of practice, mastery follows action."

YOUR PROGRESS REPORT

Write down what you learned from this chapter and what actions you plan to take. Then record what resulted from taking these actions and what you've gained.

What are three key ideas that you took away from this chapter?

1.

2.

3.

What top three actions can you take to combat a specific anxiety or fear?

1.

2.

3.

What resulted when you took these actions?

1.

2.

3.

What did you gain from taking action? What would you do differently next time?

1.

2.

3.

PART IV

Your Personal Anxieties and Fears

- See how anxiety arises from inside perfect-person traps.

- Learn how to stop feeling anxious about your imperfections.

- Exercise your free will and free yourself from needless inhibitions.

- Use an innovative PURRRRS plan to break free from anxiety restrictions.

- Discover how to liberate yourself from self-worth anxieties.

- See how to script a positive new way of being.

- Take a test and see where you stand on social anxieties.

- Follow fifty steps to leave your social anxieties behind.

- Learn how to correct mixed anxiety and depression.

- See how to stop feeling powerless over your feelings and emotions.

- Rally yourself if you lapse back to old anxiety habits.

- Fortify yourself to build resilience against needless anxiety and to prevent relapses.

CHAPTER 19

Ending Perfectionist Thinking

If you expect yourself to be flawless and make your value as a person dependent on meeting perfect standards, then you are falling into a *contingency-worth* trap. In this world of fixed convictions, it is not enough to do well; you have to do perfectly well. It's not enough to have typical performances; your performances must be exceptional. You have to avoid mistakes at all cost, lest others evaluate and reject you.

Fear of making mistakes cuts across conditions where perfectionism is maladaptive (Sassaroli et al. 2008). This negative perfectionism weaves through different forms of anxiety. Depression and perfectionism can coexist (Clara, Cox, and Enns 2007). Anger and perfectionism can coexist (Saboonchi and Lundh 2003). Substance abuse and perfectionism can coexist (Holle and Ingram 2008). Intolerance for uncertainty and perfectionism can coexist (Reuther et al. 2013). Because perfectionism weaves through so many distressing conditions, it's not surprising that perfectionism is an important transdiagnostic factor (Egan, Wade, and Shafran 2011).

If you've locked yourself into a perfectionism trap, you can use CBT to exit this self-imposed misery. CBT is effective for perfectionism (Riley et al. 2007). There is compelling evidence for favorable neural-biological changes following the use of CBT for perfectionism (Radhu et al. 2012). These favorable changes will buttress you against the fallacy that through achieving infallibility, you'll gain complete control over your emotions, others, and life.

PERFECT-PERSON TRAPS

Ordinarily, you can change perfectionist thoughts and beliefs that interfere with leading a quality life. These thoughts occur in different contexts and come in several different, overlapping forms.

Self-Perfectionism

Self-perfectionism reflects a philosophy that says, "I must behave in a certain way or I am unworthy. I must not make mistakes. I must have approval to feel worthy. I must maintain my image and appearance at all costs." Who wouldn't feel anxious under these conditions?

To question these ideas, you can focus on what you can do rather than theoretical ideas about who you should be and what you must do.

Social Perfectionism

Social perfectionism is the view that others should comply with the way you see the world. This usually backfires. Other people typically have their own notions of reality, and these notions may fit with your views only some of the time.

To build emotional tolerance, you can learn to accept—not like—that others don't have to think and feel as you do. In this enlightened state, you are likely to avoid people whose characteristics you don't like. You are likely to pick your friends among those who share your interests and values and trust. You'll feel less emotionally rattled when things don't go your way.

Learning Perfectionism

Learning perfectionism is when you are your own worst critic when it comes to learning a new skill. You may be able to accept awkwardness in others' efforts that you can't accept in yourself.

The fact is that anyone can experience awkwardness when building a new skill. Some failure is instructive. How else can you learn? Accept that learning and frustration go hand in hand, and you may feel less self-conscious when it comes time to learn something new. Instead, you may feel curious.

The Comparative Trap

The comparative trap is when you ceaselessly compare your accomplishments to other people's accomplishments and judge what you do to be less good. This view increases your risk of feeling anxious in the presence of others whom you believe are superior to you.

As an antidote to this kind of thinking, concentrate on what you can do well and let the other guys worry about their own performances.

Performance Anxiety

Performance anxiety may trap you when you believe that you must succeed in whatever you undertake. There can be no mistakes. A writer keeps revising a book. The work never gets done because it is never perfect. The inventor abandons a promising idea because she has no guarantee of success.

To exit this trap, teach yourself to recognize that the development of complex ideas and things is a process. For example, a great invention rarely starts out perfect.

You can then perform to the best of your abilities and keep chipping away until you meet reasonable-quality standards.

REQUIRING VS. ASPIRING PHILOSOPHIES

Perfectionism serves different purposes—for example, as a compensatory drive for overcoming feelings of inadequacy by establishing ironclad controls to protect against threat. However, this misguided fantasy for security and worth has a boomerang effect. Any progress you make to achieve infallibility is never enough.

If you are in a perfect-person trap you operate with a *requiring philosophy*, in which preferences for being right convert to needs, and needs to demands, and demands to coercion. Feelings of anxiety and worthlessness blend with this process. The requiring philosophy is a formula for anxiety where the threat comes from within. This philosophy has its own language, consisting of demand terms—such as "should," "ought," and "must"—and their equivalents.

In a perfect-person trap, you define yourself in terms of dichotomies: you are either right or wrong, strong or weak, good or bad. You look at things in these black-and-white terms, and these polarities fog the window through which you view reality and are formulas for distress (Egan et al. 2007). You are likely to feel threatened and anxious if you don't meet your own expectations. Now you face the task of attempting to be what you are not, where you are likely to feel anxious that whatever you do will not be good enough.

In contrast, an *aspiring philosophy* is a more flexible way of viewing life. With an aspiring philosophy, you think in terms of preferences, anticipation, wants, desires, or wishes. You assert your positive interests and desires by going after what you want.

You can strive for excellence, which means doing the best you can with the time and resources you have available. You may prefer quality performances. Who wouldn't? However, your performances do not define you as a total success or total failure!

Thinking in Terms of Preferences

By thinking in terms of preferences, you can improve your chances of developing a more relaxed and tolerant approach to life. With greater tolerance, you are likely to be more attentive to what you truly find important. You are also likely to have fewer bouts with parasitic anxieties.

EXERCISE: CONSIDER THE WORDS YOU USE

Look at the lists of words associated with these two contrasting philosophies. Which language feels more familiar to you?

Requiring Philosophy	Aspiring Philosophy
expect	desire
demand	prefer
have to	would like to
must	wish
ought	favor
should	want

If you like the feel of an aspiring philosophy, the next time you start to use a requiring-philosophy word, stop and see if you can switch it to an aspiring-philosophy word.

While there is no law that says you must choose an aspiring philosophy over a requiring philosophy, doing so is likely to have positive consequences.

Expectations Vs. Expectancies

To further help detach from perfectionist demands, consider the difference between expectations and expectancies. *Expectations* are a typical part of perfectionist thinking. Here you act as if you believe that life should, ought to, or must go as you expect. If you believe this nonsense, reality will repeatedly thwart your expectations.

In contrast, *expectancies* are probability statements. If life is filled with probabilities and only a few absolutes (like, "the sun rises in the morning"), then it makes sense to think in probability terms. You are less likely to fall into a dichotomous-thinking trap. You are more likely to feel self-assured when you have fewer unreasonable demands and unrealistic expectations to contend with. When you think in terms of expectancies, you open your mind to a range of outcomes that you may aspire to realize.

Of course, it is unlikely that anyone will achieve a purely aspiring state of mind. After all, we're all fallible. Perfect consistency is unlikely. Progress is probable.

Getting Off the Contingency-Worth Seesaw

The contingency-worth paradigm for perfectionism is *I must do what I expect of myself, or I am unacceptable.* In this conditional state of mind, you are on an emotional seesaw: up when you do well, down when you don't.

Using cognitive interventions, however, you can get off this seesaw. Here are four examples of cognitive interventions for perfectionist contingencies:

Contingency 1: "I have to be a winner." You may think that you have to win all the time, but this belief will make you feel like a loser whenever you don't measure up to your own expectations. It's important to question the idea that not winning all the time makes you a loser. It is helpful to remember that you are the same person whether or not you find yourself successful in all the big and small things that you undertake. Winning can yield advantages, but doing less well sometimes than you'd prefer makes you no more of a loser than misspelling a word makes you incompetent.

Contingency 2: "I have to be in control, or else I will feel helpless." With this contingency in place, you can make yourself feel extra anxious over the idea that without perfect self-control, you are powerless. You may also think that you can't make self-improvements unless you have all the power you think you need. But if being in perfect control is the only solution for overcoming a feeling of powerlessness, and you also believe that you are powerless to change, then how can you ever be in control? One way out of this dilemma is to accept that perfect control is a myth, that partial control is better than no control, and acceptance of what you can't control is a form of control where you've chosen reality over despair.

Contingency 3: "I must be comfortable to feel secure." If you think that to feel secure, you have to be comfortable, what happens when you start to feel uncomfortable? Will telling yourself that you must be comfortable help? You now have another dilemma. You can't escape discomfort. For example, facing uncertainty can feel uncomfortable. Conflicts are inevitable, and they can feel uncomfortable. Thus, if your freedom from anxiety depends upon consistently feeling comfortable, and some discomfort is part of living, you can't win. Accepting this reality is a step in the direction of relief from fear of discomfort.

Contingency 4: "I must have universal approval to feel worthwhile." It is usually a good idea to get along with others. Approval is beneficial. But what if you can't be loved by everyone, and yet you think you need everyone's love? This contingency for happiness is a formula for anxiety, particularly if you doubt that you can get the approval that you think you need. Preferring approval to disapproval is normal. However, you can't please everyone. Keep that in mind and you are less likely to torment yourself over what you can't control.

You may be afraid of making mistakes and try to avoid making them. You can use behavioral exposure interventions to overcome the kind of fear that you experience when you are in a situation where erring is possible.

EXERCISE: COMBAT PERFECTIONISM BY MAKING MISTAKES

To desensitize yourself to your fear of making mistakes, intentionally make some inconsequential errors. For example, in the presence of a friendly associate, get a date wrong and see what happens. Misquote the newspaper to a neighbor. Show up extra early for an appointment.

Document what happens. Are your fears realized? At worst, does someone correct you? If that happens, is it the end of the world?

Top Tip: Show Yourself a Different Movie

Long Island psychologist and couples therapist Dr. Joel Block is a strong proponent of helping people live happy and healthy lives. The author of over twenty books, including *Saving My Life: A Least Likely to Succeed Success Story*, Block gives a top tip for combatting anxiety: "If you fear a flawed performance, substitute an enlightened form of behavioral rehearsal for a perfectionist compensatory striving.

"Michael Phelps, the most medaled Olympian in history, created a video in his mind's eye and practiced it repeatedly. At his coach's urging, he practiced seeing something going wrong and coping with it. The image Phelps envisioned was seeing himself swim with his goggles filled with water. In other words, he would be swimming blind. At a competition, his coach would instruct, "Play the video," and Phelps would see himself in his mind's eye swimming blind. In fact, once it actually happened in an international competition: his goggles filled up, and he not only swam blind; he broke the world record!

"What Phelps did, using imagery as a rehearsal to manage his anxiety, has a substantial history in science. Imagery has been used to assist medically ill patients toward wellness, to speed the recovery of athletes in rehab, and in many other situations. Phelps created new neural pathways as he overcame his anxieties, and this process helped him deflate the power of his negative images. You can do the same. Rather than showing the movie that is feeding your anxiety, show a movie that shows what you fear happening but with a different ending. Picture yourself coping successfully with whatever you fear, repeat that movie in your head several times daily, and you'll find, if the event actually occurs (it usually doesn't!), that your anxiety response is going to be much reduced, or eliminated altogether."

YOUR PROGRESS REPORT

Write down what you learned from this chapter and what actions you plan to take. Then record what resulted from taking these actions and what you've gained.

What are three key ideas that you took away from this chapter?

1.

2.

3.

What top three actions can you take to combat a specific anxiety or fear?

1.

2.

3.

What resulted when you took these actions?

1.

2.

3.

What did you gain from taking action? What would you do differently next time?

1.

2.

3.

CHAPTER 20

How to Stop Inhibiting Yourself

In *The Glass Menagerie* by Tennessee Williams (1974), shy Laura Wingfield lives a quiet, isolated life with her collection of glass animals. Having a slight limp, she magnifies its significance, identifies herself with it, and limits herself because she sees herself as an unwanted invalid. Desiring love and companionship, she also fears exposing her inadequacies and getting rejected. She inhibits a normal desire because of her fear.

If, like Laura, you hold yourself back in areas where self-expression and assertion are highly appropriate, what can you do to liberate yourself? You have choices. You can do nothing and stay stuck in patterns that you want to escape but are afraid to abandon. You can wait until the time is right, but chances are you'll be waiting a long time. You can take corrective actions starting now. If it is important enough to do, avoid letting your excessive inhibitions stand in the way.

EXERCISING YOUR FREE WILL

There are two major forms of inhibitions. One is a behavioral inhibition that is visible early in life and associated with restricted exploration, stifled curiosity, avoiding uncertainties, and social anxiety. Overly inhibited young children, for example, are at elevated risk of developing social anxieties as adults (Clauss and Blackford 2012). The other is a corrective inhibition, where you intentionally allow yourself to experiment and explore as you restrain yourself from engaging in stifling inhibitions and parasitic anxieties. Indeed, it is a paradox that by learning to inhibit needless inhibitions, you can do much to liberate yourself from these emotional shackles.

Intentional acts of self-restraint are acts of free will. When you act with self-restraint, you do so knowing you could have behaved differently. For example, because you want to keep your job, you restrain your impulses to play computer games at work. You feel annoyed at your mate, but you bite your tongue to avoid a useless spat. Showing this kind of self-restraint is the mirror opposite of holding yourself back when self-assertion is appropriate. It is also different from exercising overly constrictive inhibitions.

The acronym PURRRRS stands for *pause, use your resources, reflect, reason, respond, review,* and *stabilize*. You can use the PURRRRS method to exercise your free will to reduce needless inhibitions. PURRRRS will also help you combat feelings of inadequacy associated with an inhibiting anxiety. You'll also learn to develop the kind of patience that comes from working out problems in lieu of automatically withdrawing and avoiding healthy challenges.

Pause: When you suspect that you are excessively inhibiting yourself, pause and consider what is happening. Are you feeling tense, tight, and restricted? These emotional cues can connect to inhibiting thoughts.

Use your resources: What resources can you use to resist falling down the slippery slope of inhibition? How about patience? As a start, you can agree with yourself to suspend judgment about your inhibitions until you've worked through the problem situation.

Reflect: Most excessively inhibited people are skilled at finding examples to support their inhibitory beliefs. At this stage, agree with yourself to take a self-observant view. Step back and map out your thoughts and beliefs.

Reason: You'll often find incongruities between your inhibitory beliefs and your emotional and social capabilities. Contrast your inhibitory beliefs with an adaptive perspective. First identify examples of skills showing that you possess competency (you can think; you can reason; you have accomplishments and achievements). Next, contrast examples of inhibitory thinking with these examples of competency. You now have an incongruity. Which is right? Finally, ask yourself what behavioral steps you can take to build upon your capabilities and decrease your needless inhibitions. These steps form your action plan.

Respond: Armed with a reasoned way to address your inhibitions, you now take action. You follow the steps that you outlined in your action plan.

Review: After taking action to contend with an excessively restricting inhibition, you can look at results and then decide if you can improve upon what you've done. What actions bear repeating? What seems promising that you can modify? What actions merit ditching?

Stabilize: How do you stabilize your self-improvements? Every new situation has its own unique features. By creating experiences to defuse behavioral inhibitions, you learn what you can do in a given situation. You learn how to give yourself the confidence that you can dispatch needless inhibitions.

EXERCISE: USING PURRRRS TO BATTLE INHIBITION

Write down the inhibition that you want to target. Then develop a PURRRRS plan to boost your self-reflective skills and to defeat your inhibition.

Target inhibition: _____

Your Personal PURRRRS Plan

PURRRRS	Actions
Pause: Stop and prepare for action.	
Use your resources: Apply your will and other resources to resist anxious inhibitory impulses.	
Reflect: Think about your thinking.	
Reason: Look for incongruities between your inhibitory beliefs and what you can accomplish. What new steps can you take to accomplish what you want to do?	
Respond: Put yourself through the paces of change.	
Review: Review process and make adjustments when results suggest trying another way.	
Stabilize: Persist with evolving process until parasitic inhibition is under control.	

After reading the rest of this chapter, you may want to return to this PURRRRS exercise to include other coping strategies that you've learned.

OVERCOMING INHIBITION

Live a life of overly restrictive rules, and you'll feel bound by excessive restraints. Living your life at self-restricting extremes, you've lost sight of the Aristotelian golden mean. This is the desirable range between *excesses* (when actions are driven by impulse) and *deficiencies* (when actions are driven by inhibition). Buddhist philosophy also includes the concept of the middle way.

Stepping Out of Character

You may characteristically restrict yourself too much because you are afraid of violating rules that most others would find arbitrary and excessive. You may act as if you believed that you must do nothing to bring attention to yourself. You may believe that you should do nothing that even slightly inconveniences others.

It may be time to try a stepping-out-of-character exercise. Doing this may liberate you to make reasoned rather than inhibitory judgments and decisions.

EXERCISE: TRYING SOMETHING DIFFERENT

Pretend that you are a person with fewer inhibitions. Try doing things the way this person would do them:

- The next time you go to a restaurant for breakfast and see "two eggs, any style" on the menu, order one scrambled and one fried egg.

- At lunch, order a grilled cheese sandwich with one slice of wheat and one slice of white bread.

- Wear one white and one black sock for the day.

- Visit a town where you've never been before. Ask three people for directions.

- Without making a purchase, ask for change at a convenience store.

- If you normally express yourself quietly, raise the volume.

- Go to a museum by yourself and ask total strangers what they think about the exhibits.

- Go to lunch with someone who's typically loud and boisterous. Does that person draw attention in the restaurant? Who is the attention directed toward? How does that matter?

As you do this exercise, you may want to keep a journal of the results. Review what happened. What did you learn?

By experimenting with activities that you would characteristically avoid, you position yourself to overcome inhibiting anxieties. The next time you feel a surge of inhibition and you recognize that your inhibition is unreasonable and excessive, you can remind yourself that you can overcome inhibitory feelings.

A Positive Language Experiment

Insecurity, anxiety, and inhibition typically involve negative thinking and language that support inhibition. The words you use take a leading role in how you read situations and feel, so changing your language can have a positive impact on your outlook.

If you are not in the habit of doing so, expressing yourself using positive emotional words may at first feel both uncomfortable and unnatural, but what's wrong with using positive expressions?

EXERCISE: USING POSITIVE LANGUAGE

Try reciting a list of upbeat sensory words to yourself three times a day. Recall these words in your mind before entering social situations. Use such words as "serendipitous," "soft," "pleasant," "warm," "kindly," "joyful," "happy," "mellow," "velvety," "sweet." Refer to a thesaurus for more. Practice using one or two of these words daily in conversation.

Getting over feeling uncomfortable about using positive expressions may help you build an adaptable and uninhibited outlook.

Defusing Inhibition with Humor

Humor is a promising antidote for inhibition. What can you do to tickle your funny bone when you are feeling inhibited?

- Read books by your favorite humorist.

- Watch a funny movie.

- Spend time with people who make you laugh.

- Use your imagination to turn something fearful into something hilarious.

It's hard to laugh and feel inhibited at the same time.

A Sensory Awareness Experiment

The Russian physiologist Ivan Pavlov lectured that as humans we are first connected to our environment through sensory experience. But with the evolution of language, we depart from our roots, and words increasingly substitute for sensory awareness. This separation becomes the basis for many forms of human distress (Pavlov 1941).

The gestalt therapist Fritz Perls developed a technique that is compatible with Pavlov's views. He thought people waste too much time engaging mentally in polarity conflicts, such as between good and bad. These polarities split you off from other aspects of your personality. His focus was to help people confront their conflicts, accept their experiences, and develop a healthy *gestalt*, or sense of wholeness.

Perls described a sensory awareness exercise that is worth testing (Perls, Goodman, and Hefferline 1951).

EXERCISE: PRACTICING SENSORY AWARENESS

Over the next week, take fifteen minutes a day to move about your outside environment. Observe through your senses. What do you smell, hear, feel, see, and taste? Look for sensory experiences you have not been aware of before. Preface each new sensory experience with the phrase, "Now I'm aware of..." For example, you may see a pot filled with colorful plants that you have not noticed before ("Now I am aware of a blue and gold flowerpot with red flowers"). As you pass a pizza parlor, you may smell the pizza ("Now I am aware of the scent of pizza"). You may observe the movement of a cat ("Now I'm aware of a running cat"). The clouds in the sky might change ("Now I'm aware of clouds overhead").

When you are not listening to yourself, your ears can pick up sounds that otherwise might have gone unnoticed. Your other senses are sharpened as well. Going back to your sensory roots can get you out of an inhibitory mind-set.

ASSERTING YOURSELF

Alfred Adler (1927) thought that every change brings up apprehension and fears. Fears result from how we evaluate the change. His solutions involve recognizing how you suffer interpretation errors and educating yourself to remove these errors.

The conditioned-reflex therapist Andrew Salter (1949) took a more behavioral approach to defeating inhibition. He recommended disinhibiting yourself by expressing yourself even if you insult others. He believed such actions are preferable to an obsequious, inhibited manner. Salter went on to say that if you take extreme positions that oppose your inhibitions, you are eventually likely to strike a balance. Salter is credited with starting the assertiveness movement.

Assertiveness in the aggressive sense that Salter suggests is currently out of vogue. Psychologists Robert Alberti and Michael Emmons (2008) describe *assertiveness* as self-expression directed toward equalizing relationships with others. Empathy, honesty, straightforwardness, and omitting needlessly harmful statements characterize a healthy assertive style. For example, most people regret holding back and are quite acceptant of negative results when they believe that they did the best they could; some situations won't work out, but you won't know if you don't try.

You could be both self-restrained and self-expressive at the same time. You understand the value of holding back needlessly hurtful comments, and so you act with restraint. You also understand that expressing your views is the very thing to do. A flexible balance between reasonable inhibitions and honest self-expression is a worthy antidote to inhibitions that drive anxiety and anxieties that drive inhibitions.

Top Tip: Express Yourself with Confidence

Assertiveness expert Dr. Bob Alberti is a fellow of the American Psychological Association, the author or coauthor of a half-dozen books, including *Your Perfect Right: Assertiveness and Equality in Your Life and Relationships* (which he wrote with Michael Emmons), and the editor of more than one hundred books by other psychology professionals. He shares this tip for becoming a more expressive and assertive you:

"Sweaty palms, faster heartbeat, uneasy stomach, muscle tension—life happens. Maybe it's job interviews, asking people for favors, saying no to unreasonable requests, dealing with an angry person.

"One way to deal with anxiety in such situations is to behave assertively. Express yourself. Say what you're feeling. Don't worry about saying the 'right' words. It turns out it's not so much *what* you say as *how* you say it: look directly at the other person, stand up straight, use firm but friendly gestures and facial expressions, keep your voice calm and conversational, be persistent in stating your case.

"Try this: Imagine a situation that makes you anxious—a job interview, perhaps. Picture yourself entering with a smile, shaking hands firmly, speaking clearly, feeling calm and confident, sitting up straight, making eye contact, and answering questions effectively. Go over these responses frequently before the actual event—in your mind, or with a friend, or both—until they start to feel natural. Then go out there and apply what you've learned. Your assertive action will put anxiety in the backseat, and, more often than you think, you'll come across effectively.

"Practice, practice, practice! Practice may not make perfect, but it makes better! And the practice—psychologists call it 'behavior rehearsal'—can even be in your head! Neuroscientists have found that our brains can learn about as well from imagining a scene as from living it.

"No, you won't get perfect at saying the right thing just the right way every time—nobody does—but you'll feel a lot less anxious and a lot more comfortable in most social situations. Bonus: you'll find you're much more in charge of your own life."

YOUR PROGRESS REPORT

Write down what you learned from this chapter and what actions you plan to take. Then record what resulted from taking these actions and what you've gained.

What are three key ideas that you took away from this chapter?

1.

2.

3.

What top three actions can you take to combat a specific anxiety or fear?

1.

2.

3.

What resulted when you took these actions?

1.

2.

3.

What did you gain from taking action? What would you do differently next time?

1.

2.

3.

CHAPTER 21

Overcoming Self-Anxiety

Most people spend over half their waking hours reflecting and thinking about themselves (Morin and Hamper 2012). It's what and how you think that can make a difference in the quality of your life. For example, how you think about yourself and about what you can do is central to your sense of well-being and to whether or not you suffer from anxiety.

If you worry a lot about yourself, you are likely to be excessively sensitive to threats to your sense of worth. You also are likely to exaggerate threats.

However, by addressing your needless anxieties and fears about yourself, you can forge a strong and realistic self-concept that is based on your ability to meet worthy challenges.

EXPLORING YOUR SENSE OF SELF

You sense of self may be difficult to define, but it is no illusion that you have a sense of identity and of self. You describe yourself by name. You use pronouns, such as *I, me, mine,* and *myself.* You recognize yourself in a mirror. Indeed, you can recognize early photos of yourself, even decades after they were taken (Butler et al. 2013).

In fact, your sense of self resides in separate networked regions of your brain. For example, there appear to be dominant regions of the brain for self-awareness (Craig 2009), performance monitoring (Ham et al. 2014), self-reflection (Moran, Kelley, and Heatherton 2013), self-referencing, (Abraham 2013), and cognitive reappraisal (Ochsner and Gross 2008). When networked, these parts collectively represent aspects of the self, but they are not the whole story. There is still much to learn about how we construct our self in our minds and how the brain processes self-oriented information.

Your Self-Worth

Whatever you believe about yourself represents your concept of your self. This concept may be tied to your *theory of worth*, or how you judge your general sense of self.

Do you base your self-worth on your performance, appearance, mood, or other specific factors, such as your contributions to your society? If so, you have a theory of worth that is based on contingencies. For example, with a perfectionist mind-set, if you do well, you are worthy. If you don't, you are unworthy. If your group makes *loyalty* a criterion for worth, you are worthy if you are loyal and unworthy if you fall short of this standard.

Contingency-worth theories are hotbeds for *self-anxiety*, or a general sense of uneasiness, vulnerability, and insecurity that you feel about your self. For example, if you believe that you can't measure up to your own or others' standards, you may feel anxious when you anticipate being in a situation where you may expose your vulnerabilities. When exaggerating the risk of putting yourself in an unfavorable light, you may cover up what you think you lack by even avoiding reasonable opportunities to thrive that most others would undertake.

Your Theory of Worth

When you think of your self, what comes to mind? Do you tend to think in dichotomous terms: you are good or bad, a hero or a coward, smart or dumb, worthy or unworthy? Do you think of traits, such as persistent, honest, altruistic, or competitive? Do you define your self on the basis of the clothing that you wear, neighborhood, automobile, education, ancestors' accomplishments, race, religion, or other group affiliations? Do you have core beliefs about life, politics, religion, success, and family that tend to be stable, thus giving you a sense of familiarity with your self? Do you identify your self as this combination of factors, or do you see these factors as only part of the whole you?

Depending on context, your theory of worth may vary somewhat or a lot, thus influencing how you view yourself and feel about yourself. You may view yourself as highly competent and confident in solving a relationship problem, yet you may shrivel in fear in the presence of authority or shy away from situations where you anticipate a difference of opinion. So, who is the real you?

The self is like the horizon that is constantly there but still changing. When anxieties and fears darken your horizon, move to a different spot.

Self-Concept and Anxiety

The language and narratives that you use to describe yourself can influence who you think you are and what you see as threats or opportunities. If you are inclined to view yourself as fragile and vulnerable, you are likely to experience more threats to your self-worth and a stronger need to protect yourself from real or imagined harm. In a scramble to act self-protectively, you see many worthwhile situations as risky and necessary to avoid. Sadly, your self-protectiveness is a poor security blanket. For example, by masking your anxieties and fears from others and by avoiding challenges, you are maintaining your anxieties and fears. Can you break this pattern? You bet!

AVOIDING THE CONTINGENCY-WORTH TRAP

Many in achievement-oriented cultures base their worth on successes and what others think of them. You are worthy if you do well and get approval. You are unworthy if you fall below your standards or other people criticize you. Thus, you may aspire to be a person without flaws. But as we saw in chapter 19, that is impossible.

Contingency-worth theories reflect either-or dichotomous thinking. You are either one thing or its opposite, a success or a failure. You may think, *I'm worthy because I look beautiful, I'm worthy because I contribute to my society,* or *I'm worthy because I'm wealthy.* However, what if you fall beneath your standard for worth? Over the years, you age and therefore can't maintain your original standard of beauty. Hewing to that contingency is a formula for insecurity.

A contingency-worth theory can be a foundation for self-anxiety if you believe *I'm not good enough, I'm not smart enough, I'm not confident enough,* or *I'm not attractive enough.* Putting these conditions on your self-worth amplifies your threat sensitivity and elevates your risk of experiencing more than your share of self-anxieties and fears.

A Pluralistic Theory of Self

You have many ways to define your self. You can choose to accept a contingency-worth definition. However, if your theory of worth is not working for you, exploring a pluralistic theory of self can give you a different perspective.

A pluralistic theory of self is the proposition that you are much more than your collected traits, qualities, aptitudes, and abilities. From a pluralistic view, you can't always be only one way: an anxious person or a tranquil one. Rather, you have thousands of attributes, abilities, feelings, experiences, and memories that exist within a universe of opportunities. You have the ability to read and learn. You have a broad range of skills. You can think, visualize a positive future, and profit from past experiences. You have countless experiences. You have social sensitivities. In a nutshell, you have a lot going for you. But there is more.

The roles you take are part of a pluralistic self-view. They might include father, daughter, teacher, executive, cook, or gadfly. Values add another dimension. These are the principles that guide what you consider most important and how you lead your life, and they can include responsibility, integrity, and persistence. Your cardinal attributes also stand out. They can include being extroverted or introverted, persistent, creative, witty, mathematical, musical, forceful, flexible, spiritual, grounded, autocratic, dominant, passive, compassionate, thoughtful, anxious, or athletic. Indeed, you may find as many as 17,953 different attribute possibilities listed in an unabridged dictionary (Allport and Obert 1936). A considerable number of words that describe the self, such as worthy, significant, and insignificant, are linked to social cognition. But you are even more complex than that.

Theory of Worth Vs. Theory of Self

If you are currently operating with a contingency-worth theory that feeds into feeling anxious about yourself, you may find it useful to match a contingency-worth definition against a pluralistic view of self. Here you face a paradox. If you believe that your self-worth depends upon what you do and what others think of you, but you also see yourself as a complex, multifaceted person with countless attributes and experiences, how do you reconcile these two self-views?

When you feel anxious about yourself, here is a question to consider: how can a complex, multifaceted person be worthless for making a mistake or disappointing someone or not doing as well as you might like? If you make your worth contingent on only a few of the thousands of self-attributes that make up who you are, then what is your basis for discounting the value of the rest?

There is no inflexible rule that says you have to choose between a contingency theory of worth and a pluralistic theory of self. But what makes the most sense for you to do, define yourself by a theory of worth or a theory of self?

Top Tip: Put Your Ego in Perspective

Charlottesville, Virginia author, adjunct professor, and psychotherapist Dr. Russ Grieger suggests that to avoid anxiety over your ego, you take a composite view of your self.

"Ego anxiety stems from the mistaken belief that your 'self' will be rendered bad or inadequate if you do not perform well or if others don't approve of you. You frame success and approval as not just advantageous but necessary. You make yourself anxious when you believe that either your next performance must be exceptional or you'll be damned to external worthlessness. If you fall into this trap, here are three steps to free yourself:

1. Show yourself that while your behavior and traits are definable, you are not. You act in different ways (e.g., walk, chew gum, write articles), but you are not any one of these actions. You have inner qualities (like an IQ, values, traits) and outer possessions (like a house, a body, a family). They exist, but they do not define the essence of you.

2. Show yourself that while you may rate your actions and possessions as good or bad, it is illogical to rate your whole self as either good or bad.

3. Figure out how the dots connect. Think of a circle filled with so many dots that they merge together. The circle represents all your actions, qualities, and possessions. A good dot may very well pay off, but it doesn't generalize to making you a good person. A bad dot may produce negative consequences, but it doesn't make you all bad. By separating ego (the dots) from the circle (the self), you can see that you can rate the dots. Rating the self from a biased selection of dots is arbitrary."

KELLY'S ROLE CONSTRUCTS

Personal-construct theorist George Kelly mapped how we construct reality through the scripts we follow. If a script links to problems, we can edit the script (Kelly 1955). We can do this because of our ability to anticipate what will happen next: "The world keeps on rolling on and revealing these predictions to be either correct or misleading. This fact provides the basis for the revision of constructs" (Kelly 1955, 14).

Your ability to anticipate gives you a big advantage. You can use this ability to better assert self-control, act to control the environment, respond to changing events, and initiate changes with the aim of changing your course when you think you are heading in a wrong direction.

Kelly observed that most people act like scientists. They have theories about themselves, others, and the world around them. They make observations. They gather facts. They generalize. They make predictions. But this process can be naive and flawed. For example, what happens if you repeatedly anticipate threats that do not exist?

Kelly suggests reconstructing these anticipations. For example, reconstruction can come about by debunking exaggerated expectations and creating expectancies with a better fit to reality. He thought that changes in perception come about through experimenting with new behaviors. He emphasized risk taking, adventure, and creativity. He saw personal development as a process of extending your capabilities and reorganizing what you do based upon results.

Kelly's approach applies to altering the negative evaluations and exaggerations that contribute to a concept of a vulnerable self. By acting as if you can do better, you are likely both to do better and to gain relief from self-oriented anxieties.

Establishing a New Character

Practically everyone can find scripted patterns that reflect disharmony within themselves. Kelly would say that we would be wise to change these patterns. His idea was to rewrite the negative scripts that we play, create a new narrative, practice the new script, and keep what works.

To change your anxiety-thinking script to a positive one, you can create a pretend person, give the person a name, and keep it to yourself. This pretend person can do what you've seen others do effectively in similar circumstances; such actions are likely to have a positive impact.

After giving your pretend person a name, you design a new script to describe measurable and achievable changes in your behavior. For example, instead of being tongue-tied around authority, the pretend person may speak naturally, as if talking to a friend. Instead of habitually taking blame, the pretend person assesses situations to determine where accountability lies. The pretend person accepts conflict and deals with it.

In creating your script, you can turn a contingency-worth problem into a constructive alternative. Instead of defining your worth based on contingencies, you can turn these contingencies into worthwhile goals. For example, improving your grades can remain a goal after you no longer see your self-worth as tied to making straight As. If you want to improve your relationships with the significant people in your life, work at achieving this goal. See what your pretend person can accomplish!

EXERCISE: WRITE A NEW SCRIPT

Create a new name for yourself. Keep the name a secret. (This is like an actor assuming a new identity and name for the purposes of playing a part.) As you write your script, give yourself specific instructions, including information about how the pretend person will act, speak, dress, move around, and engage in the world. Use the following steps as guidelines:

1. Describe how you tend to anticipate acting in certain situations when you feel driven by anxieties and fears. This is what you want to change. Write this in the third person (use "he" or "she").

2. Draft the new script to include the changes that you want to make. Describe what your pretend person does in targeted situations. Consider how your pretend person would act without the burden of fear: how would this person think, feel, and act differently? Describe your pretend person's approach.

3. When writing the script, define how you can have a positive impact on other people while you are advancing your own interests. Consider how your pretend person will project his or her voice, use body language, determine types of risks, and choose how to express ideas and feelings.

Test the script for about two weeks. At the end of that time, you'll have figured out what to drop, what to modify, and what feels right. If part of the role seems especially promising from the start, extend it. If part of the role falls flat, modify it or drop it.

Try it out. See what you can accomplish. If you interpret a positive change in your behavior as "faking it," your self-view could be governed by this negative interpretation. However, whatever you accomplish is within your ability to do: if you can fake acting nonanxiously, you can act nonanxiously.

YOUR PROGRESS REPORT

Write down what you learned from this chapter and what actions you plan to take. Then record what resulted from taking these actions and what you've gained.

What are three key ideas that you took away from this chapter?

1.

2.

3.

What top three actions can you take to combat a specific anxiety or fear?

1.

2.

3.

What resulted when you took these actions?

1.

2.

3.

What did you gain from taking action? What would you do differently next time?

1.

2.

3.

CHAPTER 22

From Social Anxiety to Social Confidence

You want to stop feeling self-conscious, insecure, and socially inhibited. You want to stop worrying about making social blunders and looking like a jerk. You're tired of receding into the background at social gatherings, hoping no one will see you. You're tired of your heart pounding and of feeling flush and stiff in social situations.

Can you change a pattern of social anxieties and fears to one of confident composure? Knowing what to do and taking action can help you to get past trepidations about going to weddings, joining colleagues for lunch, meeting someone whom you'd like to date, or other social-anxiety conditions that affect you. Using tested cognitive, emotive, and behavioral methods, you can face and resolve your social fears in the context where they occur.

Cognitive behavioral therapy approaches for social anxiety disabilities are highly effective (Butler et al. 2006). Neuroimaging studies show positive brain changes following the use of CBT interventions for social anxieties (Galvao-de et al. 2013).

SOCIAL ANXIETIES AND FEARS

Even the most confident people can sometimes experience stage fright. Social anxieties and fears are more than just getting the jitters, however. You dread the thought of getting tongue-tied, socially fumbling, turning red, boring people, or looking like a fool. You attend a social event, and it feels like a torture chamber. Lacking social confidence, you may avoid answering your phone or signing up for a course of study because you feel uncomfortable around new people. You may feel awkward making small talk. When asked to make a comment, you choke and try to get it over with as quickly as you can.

The psychological core of social anxiety includes at least three primary parts. You feel out of emotional control in the social situations where you feel fearful. You anticipate being evaluated, judged, disapproved of, and rejected. You dread the unpleasant physical and emotional sensations that you anticipate will come about in social situations that you fear. With all this mental and emotional commotion, you are likely to avoid social circumstances where you anticipate feeling self-conscious and awkward.

Control is a transdiagnostic factor that cuts across different social anxieties and is a prime target for cognitive behavioral therapy (Gallagher, Naragon-Gainey and Brown 2014). For example, if you believed that you could exercise control over yourself, accept yourself with or without the approval of a few others, and tolerate the physical sensations of tension, you might test social situations that you'd normally avoid or suffer through. This *assertion of control* coping belief can dramatically ease your social anxieties and fears.

Social Phobia Facts

If you suffer from a painful social-evaluation anxiety, you're hardly alone. The lifetime prevalence for people suffering from severe social anxieties and fears is 12.1 percent of the US population (Kessler et al. 2005). However, the real numbers are likely to be higher. Many more people may restrict their lives out of fear of offending anyone, looking bad, or engendering disapproval for very trivial matters. Indeed, many who suffer from social anxieties mask them to avoid embarrassment.

Social anxieties and fears typically start in childhood or during adolescence (Rosellini et al. 2013). In some studies, men and women are about equally affected (Beesdo et al. 2007). In others, women are more likely to be socially phobic (Crome, Baillie, and Taylor 2012). Women are more likely to blame themselves for their social phobia problem, while men are more likely to blame others and use alcohol and drugs to medicate their anxieties (Xu et al. 2012).

When severe, social anxieties can strongly influence your choice of mate, career, recreational opportunities, and the quality of your life. Males with social phobias tend to marry later and artificially limit their occupational opportunities. Social phobias can place limits on a woman's career and often on the selection of a mate: a woman with social phobias tends to settle rather than select.

Coexisting Conditions

Social fears and anxiety practically always have coexisting complications. Depression is common (Ingram et al. 2005). Perfectionism is common (Ashbaugh et al. 2007). Alcohol and drug abuse are common (Baillie and Sannibale 2007).

SOCIAL ANXIETY AND YOU

Along with the physical survival circuit that New York University neuroscientist Joseph LeDoux (2012) identified, you have a parallel social brain circuitry with elaborate connections between different brain regions that process socially relevant information, such as facial expressions, social emotions, and social interactions (Li, Mai, and Liu 2014). Because of these structures, our natural ability to be conditioned, and a long developmental process, we are exposed to extensive social conditioning where we learn to conform to social rules, norms, and responsibilities. Through this lengthy process, some of us become social casualties by learning to worry too much about what others think and to needlessly restrict what we do because of excessive anxieties about social censure (Knaus 2000).

Our lives are significantly shaped by our beliefs and emotions, and so we expect ourselves to feel and act in certain ways based on the social context we are in. However, at least some of our excess painful social emotions (such as social anxiety, shame, embarrassment, self-consciousness) are associated with false expectations and beliefs. When belief-based anxieties and fears weave through your social life, you have a significant challenge to get beyond these interferences if you choose to do and feel better in social settings.

Do you have social anxieties and fears that merit correcting? You can take a test to see. The following social-fears inventory samples thoughts, feelings, and actions commonly experienced by people with social anxieties and fears. Use this inventory to boost your awareness of your own social anxieties and fears. Then work to reduce the ones that are the most debilitating.

EXERCISE: TAKING INVENTORY OF YOUR SOCIAL FEARS

Instructions: Rate each statement on a scale of 1 to 5, according to how well the statement describes you: 1 equals "never like me," 2 equals "rarely like me," 3 equals "sometimes like me," 4 equals "often like me," and 5 equals "practically always like me."

1. "I feel uptight meeting someone I don't know."	1	2	3	4	5
2. "I'm afraid of making a fool of myself in public."	1	2	3	4	5
3. "I have very little to offer others."	1	2	3	4	5
4. "Others are more sociable than I am."	1	2	3	4	5
5. "If people really knew me, they wouldn't like me."	1	2	3	4	5

6.	"When someone looks in my direction, I look away."	1	2	3	4	5
7.	"I'm afraid I'll make a mistake in front of other people."	1	2	3	4	5
8.	"I feel insecure about my social abilities."	1	2	3	4	5
9.	"My conversations feel strained."	1	2	3	4	5
10.	"I am poor at making small talk."	1	2	3	4	5
11.	"I worry about upcoming social events."	1	2	3	4	5
12.	"I feel intimidated in the presence of authority."	1	2	3	4	5
13.	"I believe that others think I'm weird or stupid."	1	2	3	4	5
14.	"I worry too much about what others think of me."	1	2	3	4	5
15.	"I'm afraid to answer the telephone."	1	2	3	4	5
16.	"I worry about going into a public bathroom."	1	2	3	4	5
17.	"I'm afraid of showing fear in a social setting."	1	2	3	4	5
18.	"I worry about what other people think of me."	1	2	3	4	5
19.	"I feel very ill at ease around people I don't know well."	1	2	3	4	5
20.	"I'm afraid of others seeing me afraid."	1	2	3	4	5
21.	"I feel self-conscious about my appearance."	1	2	3	4	5
22.	"I feel uncomfortable eating alone in restaurants."	1	2	3	4	5
23.	"I feel anxious entering a room with people already seated."	1	2	3	4	5
24.	"I'm afraid of criticism."	1	2	3	4	5
25.	"I feel embarrassed when I attract attention in a group."	1	2	3	4	5
26.	"I freeze up when I'm around attractive people."	1	2	3	4	5
27.	"I feel anxious if a conversation slows down."	1	2	3	4	5
28.	"I feel self-conscious when standing in line."	1	2	3	4	5

29. "I fear going to formal social events."	1	2	3	4	5
30. "I have more courage after a few drinks (or getting high)."	1	2	3	4	5
31. "I don't match up to other people's standards."	1	2	3	4	5
32. "I fade into the background in group settings."	1	2	3	4	5
33. "I stumble over my words talking to people I don't know well."	1	2	3	4	5
34. "I'll cross the street to avoid saying hello to an acquaintance."	1	2	3	4	5
35. "I experience terror at the thought of speaking before a group."	1	2	3	4	5
36. "I want to hide when people I'm with draw attention to themselves."	1	2	3	4	5

Statements rated 4 or 5 suggest a problem area for you. If you rated ten or more items as 4 or 5, you could have a general social anxiety issue to resolve. However, its something you can address. The core transdiagnostic issues may be as straightforward as anxiety over feeling out of control, evaluation anxiety, or anxiety over feeling awkward and fearful. By overcoming a core feature of social anxiety, such as evaluation anxiety, you may teach yourself to feel at ease in social situations.

You face a special challenge when you have social omissions in your life. You may be missing out on opportunities to establish desired social relationships, pick up on positive social cues, make community contributions, and follow a satisfactory career track. An anxiety-avoidance process can be so automatic that your discomfort-dodging efforts are obscured from view as they are silently woven into the fabric of your life.

Using your personal observations, an examination of social omissions in your life, and the results of the inventory, what is your most significant social anxiety or fear? Write it down. Work at whittling it down.

After you've worked for a while to reduce your social anxieties, retake the inventory to check your progress.

SOCIAL AWKWARDNESS

Some people suffer from social awkwardness, and because of this, they often procrastinate by diverting themselves to safer behaviors and situations. Social awkwardness can take many forms.

• *Tom and Bob's Story*

Tom attended a New Year's party with his friend Bob. Neither felt comfortable about striking up conversations with women. But they were quite comfortable communicating with each other.

Tom saw Sally with a group of women and found her very appealing. He thought about going over to her. To boost his courage, he slugged down a few drinks. He thought, *I need a few drinks to loosen up.* Then he did a hesitation waltz. Later, he commiserated with Bob about why women like Sally are unapproachable. At the end of the evening, he and Bob left the party entangled in an inebriated conversation about why women should approach men.

• *June's Story*

June has a warm, personable quality and feels at ease meeting new people. Despite her comfort with meeting and talking to people in social situations, June has an extreme public-speaking anxiety. Because she is afraid to speak before staff and customer groups, she refuses job promotions. She imagines herself turning red, becoming tongue-tied, and then running from the stage in disgrace. She says she'd rather spend a year in a dungeon than deliver a talk.

• *Don's Story*

Don and Ellen have an intimate date at their favorite restaurant. Ellen feels happy about the occasion and is animated and expressive. Don finds her too loud. He believes that she must be disturbing the other patrons. He criticizes Ellen for her loudness. Ellen suggests that he has a warped sense of values: she's the one he's going home with, not the strangers at the next table.

What do Tom, Bob, June, and Don have in common? Each acts self-consciously. Each expects to be evaluated. Each expects rejection. Each feels unpleasant physical fear sensations associated with social anxiety.

Top Tip: Stop Paying the Toll Twice

Atlanta psychotherapist Ed Garcia has a useful way to look at social anxiety. He sees this form of anxiety as paying the toll twice, both before the bridge and at the booth:

"Say you are anxious about attending a friend's wedding because you fear feeling out of place. Indeed, when you go to the wedding, you feel uncomfortable, out of place, and you retreat into the background. In this example, one cost is the anxiety you feel in anticipation of the event. The other cost is the fear you experience at the wedding.

"Learning to overcome anxiety over fear would eliminate the first toll. Before the toll, you can examine the reasons why you would feel out of place. You might start with a definition of *being out of place*. Here the idea is to eliminate the first toll.

"At the wedding, questioning and defusing the idea that you are out of place would go far to limit or eliminate the second toll. You could go still further if, when at the wedding, you introduce yourself to at least three people whom you do not know and talk to three people whom you do know. This form of exposure is a great way to overcome a fear of being present at a social gathering.

"With both threats gone, you might even have a good time."

FIFTY WAYS TO LOSE YOUR SOCIAL ANXIETIES

Some socially fearful people see themselves as intruders who are worthy of scorn. Fearing to displease, members of this group make unobtrusive entries and exits. So what can you do if you find yourself in this social and emotional stew? Here are fifty ways to combat your social anxieties:

Keep fighting fear. Fear of fear feeds on itself. Plan to survive this temporary discomfort. You'll find that you can survive it. Emotional tolerance is a prelude to feeling more comfortable with yourself in social situations.

Maintain perspective. Avoid focusing on your fears. Instead, ask others questions about themselves. You'll find that people are more than happy to talk about themselves.

Watch the worry. You fret about possibly acting inept. Correct this worry by instructing yourself to suspend judgment. Then act as if you were capable of communicating well with most others.

Give up playing Nostradamus. Predicting the world will crash down on you if you make a social blunder is an imaginary crisis. The anxiety from such false predictions is real enough. But you can work on changing your crooked thinking.

Avoid anticipatory anxiety. If you catastrophize about future dangers to your ego, picture yourself breaking a magnifying glass, and then imagine that your catastrophizing vision is shattered.

Level your language. Hyperbole, such as "I will disgrace myself forever if I make a social misstep," is an egregious overgeneralization. Intentionally make a minor misstep to show yourself that it's not the end of the world.

Beware of your definitions. Define a type of social event as a staging ground for looking like a fool, and you are likely to feel the way that you think. Redefine the event in a more positive light, and you will feel better.

Accept feeling awkward. Your feelings may be factual, but they are not the same as facts. If you're anxious about being socially awkward, realize that some people will find your manner charming. Try to take an "it is as it is" acceptance view.

Handle self-handicapping. Don't avoid a social gathering with the excuse that you will fail. Instead, imagine yourself cordially communicating.

Defeat your needless inhibitions. Practice doing something as basic as introducing yourself to people in a group.

Temper your timidity. Mingle softly rather than not at all.

Pen yourself in. Instead of waiting for someone to rescue you, push yourself to participate.

Keep it light. You don't have to make all brilliant remarks.

Bring yourself into the fold. Make a comment about something in the immediate area, such as the weather.

Address your ambivalence. Asking yourself *Should I or should I not say something?* is a formula for letting a conversation float past you. Assume that you should, and you are likely to be right.

Think less doubtfully. Abandon second-guessing yourself about what you should say. When in doubt, speak up.

Don't let your mind go blank. You can always say, "Hello."

Retreat from rejection. Fear of rejection is ordinarily a fictional fear. If someone justifiably rejects an idea of yours, you can still accept the parts of your idea that remain valid.

Use bashfulness as a positive signal. Instead of looking aloof, look at others as potential friends.

Manage your modesty. Get into the habit of daily sharing a positive attribute that characterizes you. You may blush less.

Watch your wariness. Don't take a backseat. Assume that some of the people whom you meet will be friendly. See if you can find them.

Accept feeling shy. If you are naturally shy, you won't eliminate this natural tendency. However, you can choose to manage your shyness. Try to discover other people's special interests by asking them questions. Do this and you may be seen as a brilliant conversationalist, even if you say little about yourself.

You don't have to be bold. Try communicating in a nonassertive, low-key way.

Don't expect immediate jubilance. If you warm to new social situations slowly, know that you are not alone and not odd.

Avoid blaming your amygdala. Social anxieties correlate with a sensitive amygdala. Nevertheless, you can buffer yourself from needless stress by habituating to it. That means practice, practice, practice communicating to others until you are no longer afraid.

Downplay listening to your heart. Attending to your heartbeat shifts your focus from what you are doing to how tense you feel. Participate. Your heart will take care of itself.

Mind your body language. Habitually gaze downward and you'll look insecure. Hold your head up. Glance around without staring. This signals confidence.

Nod your head "yes." Nodding signals approval. Most people like approval.

Try to smile. Think of something pleasing and let your smile extend from the thought.

Don't read too much into facial expressions. Assumptions about the causes and meanings of others' facial expressions are risky. We do have an inborn tendency to read faces, but not all faces are easy to read.

Attend to the facts. Shift from self-absorbing thoughts to objective observation of what is going on. Respond based on an objective awareness.

Reevaluate. To avoid rejection, you believe you must make a great first impression. Plan to make a reasonable impression, and let the chips fall where they may.

Ditch your false expectations. You don't need to be the life of the party if that is not your style.

Flip things around. If you fear total rejection, so you wither in silence in the corner, instead pretend that you'll get a million dollars to engage 10 percent of the time. I'll bet you can do it.

Don't think you must dominate. Show interest. Share a few thoughts. Let others talk. Put in your two cents' worth when a topic appeals to you.

Prepare to be pleasantly surprised. You may make serendipitous connections with people.

Don't wait to say only perfect things. Accept the concept of the cocktail party syndrome. People will rarely stay on topic and will invariably introduce their own agendas into a discussion.

Avoid conditionals for socializing. Waiting to feel comfortable before venturing out rarely works well. It's a form of procrastinating. Test the waters and see if social comfort follows.

Quell your self-consciousness. You are probably more aware of your state of mind than anyone else is.

Separate anxiety from context. If you act socially fearful in some situations but not others, how does what you tell yourself differ in these contexts?

Challenge feeling inferior. Instead of concentrating on what you think you lack, play on the strengths that you have.

Exercise your strongest social skills. List what they are. Use one each time you are part of a social gathering.

Ditch the shame. You're not globally worthless for being you. You just think you're something that you are really not.

Derail irrational guilt. It's silly to condemn yourself for errors that only you observe.

Speak up. As you practice speaking up, it gets easier.

Don't defect-detect. For every fault you find in yourself, find a positive attribute that others may observe.

Don't be coy. Evasiveness is likely to bring negative attention.

Think ahead. Plan to live through social tensions. Eventually you'll have fewer to live through.

Resist withdrawing into a bottle of wine. Alcohol-dulled senses are a staging ground for problems and for tensions that are catalysts for further drinking.

Realize you can't win them all. Nobody is a universal crowd-pleaser.

PEERING INTO THE LOOKING GLASS

Your social evaluation anxieties and fears are about you and what you think about yourself and your public image. However, you may also believe that others see you as you see yourself. This is the looking-glass effect (Cooley 1902). If you read too much negativity into social situations, your beliefs about what you think others are thinking can reflect your anxious expectations.

You can make reasonable guesses about how other people think and feel, their intentions, and what motivates them. Being able to infer other peoples' desires, emotions, and intentions is called *theory of mind* (Krause et al. 2012). Theory of mind also takes into account that some people have interests, beliefs, and motives that are different from yours and different from what you expect them to be.

Rather than embrace the looking-glass effect, you may correctly infer that some people think differently from what you expect them to think. With that perspective, you may be less inclined to jump to conclusions about what other people think of you. Instead, by exploring where you may be right, wrong, or unsure about others' impressions of you, you can stop looking through a distorted looking glass and see more clearly through the lens of reality.

CONTESTING AWFULIZING ABOUT SOCIAL ANXIETIES

You can increase social anxiety by using dramatic language, such as the words "terrible" or "unbearable," to tell yourself how you feel about an upcoming event or about something that you did already. In this awfulizing mind-set, your discomfort is "horrible." Your performance was "awful." However, sometimes the situation is not even close to being that bad.

You can use Albert Ellis's ABCDE method (see chapter 11) to overcome anxiety thinking that includes awfulizing. As an example, this ABCDE chart uses a substandard musical performance before an audience.

An ABCDE Resolution for Awfulizing a Substandard Performance

Adversity or activating event: Giving a substandard musical performance.
Reasonable beliefs about the event: "I'd like to have done better, but you can't win them all." Variability—not perfection—typifies life.
Emotional and behavioral consequences: Disappointment and unhappiness with the result. Review feedback and take advantage of the information to improve future performances.
Awfulizing beliefs about the event: "This is awful." "I'm a failure." "People hate me." "I'll never live this down."
Emotional and behavioral consequences: Self-loathing, anxiety, avoidance of future musical performances.

Disputing awfulizing beliefs:

Disputing starts with the assumption that it is beneficial to give above-average performances. The following disputation addresses four awfulizing beliefs:

1. Is the situation as awful as you think? Answer: If "awful" means 100 percent bad, can you imagine a situation that would be worse? Probably. You could have gone blind during the presentation. Your local newspaper could have carried a front-page headline saying that you did a miserable job. Recognizing that worse things could have happened can give you some much-needed perspective. Perhaps your situation may be tough to swallow, but it's not worth double-troubling yourself over.

2. Does your belief that you failed have empirical validity? Answer: The conclusion that you failed is an extension of *have-to-thinking* where, based upon a single performance, you are either a success or a failure as a person. Making this claim is ludicrous. It suggests that this one event marks you one way forever, but people can improve and do better if they work at it.

3. Does your belief that people hate you for your performance have validity? Answer: Taking a looking-glass approach and believing that all others share the same views as you do about yourself suggest that you have extraordinary powers, which you probably don't have. One performance—whether perfect or imperfect—doesn't define you.

4. Does your belief—*I'll never live this down*—seem reasonable? Answer: Concluding that you'll be remembered for this event for as long as you live suggests that what you did was so memorable that, thirty years later, someone might approach you to say, "Aren't you the one who gave that below-average musical performance?" What are the odds of that happening?

Effects of disputes: Disappointment over the performance. Acceptance of reality that public performances can be variable. A big reduction in awfulizing and related negative thinking. A willingness to work hard on your music and to perform in public again.

You can use the ABCDE method to combat awfulizing or any other irrational belief that fuels your social anxiety.

EXERCISE: ABCDE PRACTICE FOR SOCIAL ANXIETY

Describe your adversity or activating situation (a social event that will take place or has already taken place). Next, identify and list your reasonable beliefs about the event and the emotional and behavioral consequences of having these beliefs. Then, write down your anxiety beliefs and the emotional and behavioral consequences of having these beliefs. Next, dispute your anxiety beliefs and record the effects.

Your ABCDE Resolution for an Irrational Social-Anxiety Belief

Adversity or activating event:
Reasonable beliefs about the event:
Emotional and behavioral consequences of reasonable beliefs:
Anxiety beliefs about the event:
Emotional and behavioral consequences of anxiety beliefs:
Disputing anxiety beliefs:
Effects of disputes:

YOUR PROGRESS REPORT

Write down what you learned from this chapter and what actions you plan to take. Then record what resulted from taking these actions and what you've gained.

What are three key ideas that you took away from this chapter?

1.

2.

3.

What top three actions can you take to combat a specific anxiety or fear?

1.

2.

3.

What resulted when you took these actions?

1.

2.

3.

What did you gain from taking action? What would you do differently next time?

1.

2.

3.

CHAPTER 23

Coping with Mixed Anxiety and Depression

Do you feel like you are going through life mired in misery? Do you see yourself as a poster child for Murphy's law, where if something can go wrong, it will go wrong? Do you spend a lot of time either worrying or in a depressive funk? Perhaps you suffer from mixed anxiety and depression.

When anxiety and depression combine, you may feel distraught and think, *I feel like a hopeless mess.* Your tolerance for inconvenience and discomfort is likely to be unusually low. If left unaddressed, mixed anxiety and depression can linger. That doesn't have to be. (For more on how to cope with depression, see *The Cognitive Behavioral Workbook for Depression*, listed in suggested reading.)

Whether you seek professional help, engage in self-help, or do both, it is useful for you to know that you can address anxiety and depression simultaneously with evidenced-based methods. You have reason to be optimistic. This chapter will first explore research findings on mixed anxiety and depression. It will then help you work on recognizing and combatting powerlessness thinking in anxiety and depression.

RESEARCH FINDINGS ON MIXED ANXIETY AND DEPRESSION

If you suffer from a mixed anxiety and depression, you are not alone. This combination is common (Kessler et al. 2011). Co-occurrences range from 50 percent to 80 percent (Watson and Kendall 1989; Gorwood 2004; Das 2013). Depression appears to contribute to an increased overall sense of distress (Malyszczak et al. 2006).

When anxiety and depression are both present, anxiety usually comes first; 57 percent of people report having anxiety first and 18 percent report having depression first (Lamers et al.

2011). But regardless of which came first, you can develop the use of CBT methods to gain relief from both conditions (Norton, Hayes, and Hope 2004).

Actions to reduce anxiety can carry over to reduce depression. For example, CBT and related evidence-based methods appear effective for people with depression and anxiety in medical settings (Campbell-Sills et al. 2012). If you have a mixed anxiety and depression, by acting against your anxiety, you may not have to deal directly with an accompanying depression (Fergus et al. 2013). If you also suffer from panic, neither anxiety nor depression need impede coping with that condition (Allen et al. 2010).

Bibliotherapy is helpful to a subgroup of people with depression (Gregory et al. 2004). If you specifically address depression, you can use CBT methods to effect changes in higher brain functions that are associated with a reduction in depression (Goodapple et al. 2004).

CONFRONTING POWERLESSNESS THINKING

Anxieties differ in terms of their form and context. There are also different forms of depression, such as atypical depressions, chronic low-grade depressions, seasonal depressions, major depressions, and bipolar depressions. Some depressions follow stresses. Regardless of the type of mixed anxiety and depression you experience, you will usually find some co-occurring distortions in your thinking, such as powerlessness thinking. By changing this thinking, you may decrease both anxiety and depression.

Again, powerlessness thinking is the belief that you have no control over your emotions or yourself. In this state of mind, real or imagined bad situations become worse. You worry. Your future looks gloomy. You fear that your misery will linger. You feel upset over feeling upset. You act like you believe you are doomed. You feel like giving up. If you stick to these fatalistic views, you risk amplifying your feelings of misery.

The founder of individual psychology, Alfred Adler, said, "A person does not change his behavior pattern but turns, and twists, and distorts his experiences until they fit it" (Adler 1927, 11). If joint parasitic anxieties and depression keep coming back, you might believe that you can't change, and you can fall into a pessimistic procrastination trap where you never try.

If you think you can't act, you won't act. It's not that you can't teach yourself to think and act differently; it's that you won't, because you think you can't. Although it is true that some circumstances are beyond your control, to quote an old Chinese proverb, "You can't prevent the birds of sorrow from flying over your head, but you can prevent them from building nests in your hair."

Examining Powerlessness Thinking

Normal human suffering exists. The loss of a child, job, or relationship tragically is as it is. You regret what happened, and you are powerless to change it. At these times, you may experience a double trouble of distress, where you lament over lamenting. You may view yourself as powerless to stop feeling depressed, but you can change this thinking. Coming to terms with what has happened involves developing a sense of acceptance. In time, you can turn the jolt of a loss into a sad remembrance.

Having solutions available and using them are two different things, however. When anxious, you may procrastinate on testing promising solutions. You may tell yourself that you are too overwhelmed. When powerlessness thinking dominates, you may not want to try. But thinking you are powerless to change doesn't make that true.

Does it help to look for incongruities in your thinking? For example, you may think that you are powerless to cope, but can you think of a time when you coped effectively and thought of events differently? If so, the fact that you can change your thinking suggests that you can't be powerless over your thoughts.

You can feel powerless over your emotions when you believe you are under the thumb of outside forces that you can't control: "Jack made me mad." But if Jack makes you mad, and you can't control Jack, what can you do? You can own responsibility for your part of the problem: What do you tell yourself about Jack's behavior that evokes anger? What are the flaws in your thinking?

Acceptance and Powerlessness Thinking

A cat may get depressed, but doesn't succumb to powerless thinking about that depression or use it as the basis for judging its own value as a cat. When you are depressed, though, you may think of yourself as powerless to act to improve your future. This powerlessness thinking reinforces your depression, and you continue to think of yourself as powerless to act.

However, you can tell yourself that your thoughts are just thoughts. Some have negative, exaggerated meanings. They can surface in different forms.

EXERCISE: USING THE FLIP TECHNIQUE

Use a flip technique to promote a realistic new perspective. For example, if you can learn new ways to fix a broken vase, you are not powerless. If you can learn to think reflectively about your thinking, you are not very powerless.

Is it possible for you to see powerlessness thoughts as dust balls that you are sweeping out the door? Can you imagine yourself throwing lightning bolts at these thoughts, and destroying them?

By flipping things in your mind, you may come to see that the feeling of being powerless is a temporary state. If you have the power to create fearsome images, you can use imagery to alter powerlessness thinking. Although your thoughts may appear like dark clouds on the horizon, you can judge them without judging yourself.

You may believe that you are helpless to change even though you have evidence that you can make voluntary changes. How do you reconcile this incongruity? Perhaps the answer is to recognize that you can change unwanted parts of your thoughts, feelings, and actions even if changing is difficult.

Using the PURRRRS Method

You can use the PURRRRS method introduced in chapter 20 to create a plan to target powerlessness thinking that coexists with mixed anxiety and depression. Here's how:

Pause: If you are feeling powerless to change, take time out to work out this problem.

Use your resources: Put yourself into a problem-solving mind-set. The problem, in this case, is powerlessness thinking. Write out your thoughts or record them using a tape recorder so that you can review them.

Reflect: Look at or listen to your recorded thoughts, and then think about your thinking. What part of this thinking represents an assumption? For example, do you tell yourself that you can do nothing to improve your ability to cope? Does this translate into a core belief that you are powerless to change? If so, then move on to reasoning it out.

Reason: Look for exceptions to powerlessness thinking. Have you ever thought of yourself as powerless and then found something you could do to make a difference? Do you have the power to accept reality even though you may not like it?

Respond: What steps can you now take to deal with powerlessness thinking? What step will you take first? What step will you take next? Can you act to change your thinking through doing an ABCDE analysis (see chapter 11)?

Review: What if you devise a good plan and then you procrastinate? When you are engaged in this behavioral procrastination process, does powerlessness thinking contribute to subverting persistence? For example, is it that you expect yourself not to finish, and then you do what you expect? But how can you be powerful enough to prepare, to start, to move forward, but not powerful enough to finish? This type of review can be revealing. Now armed with this new information, reconsider what is happening. Try again.

Stabilize: Routinely take self-directed efforts to challenge powerlessness thinking in all its forms. Review what works for you, and redo it. Practice, practice, practice strengthening your reason to buffer yourself against the fictions of powerlessness thinking.

EXERCISE: USING PURRRRS TO COMBAT POWERLESSNESS THINKING

Use the PURRRRS system to target your own form of powerlessness thinking.

Write down the specific thinking pattern that you want to target. Then develop a PURRRRS plan to defeat it.

Target thinking: _____

Your Personal PURRRRS Plan

PURRRRS	Actions
Pause: Stop and prepare for action.	
Use your resources: Apply your will and other resources to resist impulses to capitulate to powerlessness thinking.	
Reflect: Think about what is happening.	
Reason: Think it through.	
Respond: Put yourself through the paces of change.	
Review: Review your process and make adjustments when results suggest trying another way.	
Stabilize: Persist with this evolving process until powerlessness thinking is under control.	

Top Tip: How to Talk and Walk Your Way Out of Anxiety

Dr. Clifford N. Lazarus, multimodal therapist, author of *Don't Believe It for a Minute: Forty Toxic Ideas That Are Driving You Crazy*, and the cofounder of the Lazarus Institute in Skillman, New Jersey, describes two common thinking errors that occur in both anxiety and depression. Lazarus shares this tip:

"As is often the case with depression, it is challenging to talk yourself out of anxiety. To truly conquer a mixed anxiety and depression, you need to take specific steps, such as recognizing and combatting two common thinking errors. As anxiety often precedes a major depression, I'll tell how to combat anxiety before it spreads into depression.

"Anxious people greatly overestimate the chances of a dreaded event happening and the seriousness of the consequences of the bad event if it actually happens. First, anxious people often confuse low possibility calamities (i.e., very unlikely bad events) with high probability occurrences (i.e., very likely events). In other words, they confuse the possible with the probable. The second common cognitive error is to overestimate the impact of bad events. In other words, anxious people usually believe that if something bad happens, it will produce a dramatic or even devastating consequence that might be too much to handle.

"Once you contain and correct these mental miscalculations, you can more easily begin to face and overcome the situations that trigger your anxiety. Indeed, exposure to anxiety triggers is the most important part of the anxiety solution.

"To understand why exposure is such a key part to this process, it helps to think of anxiety as a *psychological allergy*. If someone suffers from environmental allergies (like pollen, ragweed, or pet dander), it's because his or her immune system is overly sensitive to those triggers (technically called *allergens*). Instead of having a minor reaction or no reaction when exposed to certain allergens, an allergy sufferer's immune system launches a dramatic reaction resulting in the misery of an allergy attack.

"In anxious people, it's not their immune systems that overreact to the trigger of a psychological allergen (some perceived threat or danger) but a vulnerability in their nervous systems, which often leads to the misery of anxiety. And just as allergy sufferers can be successfully desensitized by exposure to gradually increasing doses of the very stuff they're allergic to, people who suffer from the psychological allergy of anxiety can be desensitized, too.

"You can help yourself to stop overreacting by gradually exposing yourself to the very situations that evoke your anxiety. For example, if you feel anxious about making a mistake, intentionally make mistakes under controlled conditions. As with allergy desensitization, over time your nervous system tones down and eventually stops overreacting to the stuff that used to set off an anxiety reaction."

YOUR PROGRESS REPORT

Write down what you learned from this chapter and what actions you plan to take. Then record what resulted from taking these actions and what you've gained.

What are three key ideas that you took away from this chapter?

1.

2.

3.

What top three actions can you take to combat a specific anxiety or fear?

1.

2.

3.

What resulted when you took these actions?

1.

2.

3.

What did you gain from taking action? What would you do differently next time?

1.

2.

3.

CHAPTER 24

Preventing Anxiety and Fear from Coming Back

However great your progress, anxiety thinking and negative feelings may not entirely disappear. You lose a few nights of sleep, and an old maladaptive anxiety habit can creep back.

However, lapses don't have to be as intense, durable, and frequent as they were before. You can recover more quickly. If you are not perfectly consistent in managing your worries and troubles, you don't have to look at yourself or the situation negatively. As the saying goes, if you fall off a horse, get back on again.

When it comes to reversals, it helps to look at the big picture. With a little perspective, you can see that you can avoid double troubles over lapsing and relapsing if you keep yourself from magnifying setbacks into catastrophes. You also can see that you have cognitive, emotive, and behavioral tools to assert control over new or older anxieties. You can see that you can tolerate tensions, which is not the same as liking them. And most importantly, you can see that life is more than just contesting anxieties. It's what you choose to make it. This big-picture thinking gives you a legitimate form of control over anxieties if they recur.

If you assume that change is a process and not an event, it is easier to accept the ups and downs of self-improvement and personal growth. Looking at change this way is far less taxing than thinking that if you slide back, everything you've done so far is worthless.

Each new anxiety event gives you an opportunity to hone your cognitive, emotional-tolerance, and behavioral skills. But you don't have to wait for anxiety to spontaneously recur in order to practice. You can use these skills regularly to actualize your finest qualities.

RALLY YOURSELF

Here are five quick steps to rally yourself against an emerging anxiety. You can use them in any order:

Review the key ideas, action plans, and exercise sections in each chapter of this book. This is a quick way to access what you found most important to think about and to do. As a maintenance measure, review this written record whenever you face an anxiety situation. As a prevention measure, review this record monthly.

Deal with double troubles. When anxieties and fears return, double troubles typically follow. This secondary distress comes in different forms: blaming yourself for backsliding, worrying about worrying, feeling disturbed about feeling disturbed, and getting depressed about feeling depressed. You'll do much to prevent adding to your distress if you deal with these double troubles when they arise.

Do a BASIC-ID review for diagnostic, prescriptive, and maintenance purposes. What's going on with each of the modalities? If there is a hot spot, ask yourself what you can do about it. Then, act! The system's pioneer Arnold Lazarus (1992) recommends a monthly BASIC-ID review as an early warning system (see chapter 18).

Invoke PURRRRS to engage your self-observant abilities. When you control your anxiety through PURRRRS, you position yourself to control the outcome (see chapters 20 and 23).

Use your ABCDEs to challenge anxiety thinking. As you practice the ABCDE method (see chapters 11, 16, and 22), you will get better at using it. As you get more skilled, you will find less need to use it.

LIGHTEN YOUR ALLOSTATIC LOAD

Normal conditions of daily living involve stresses and adjustments to stresses. You can't escape it. For example, when you jump into the ocean for a swim, your body adjusts to the change. When you are stuck in traffic and running behind schedule, you feel frustrated. Your body adjusts to the frustration and then to relief when traffic suddenly starts to move.

Rockefeller University professor Bruce McEwen (2006) studies the relationship between the mind and the whole body to show how stress affects this interactive system. He is specifically interested in the *allostatic load factor* in health and disease. This is the cumulative wear and tear on your body from repeated changes and readjustments to various stressful social, personal, and environmental events (McEwen and Wingfield 2003). By reducing needless stresses, you can improve your health. That's a big-picture benefit.

Allostatic load theory links higher stress to disease, and poor coping predicts a higher allostatic load (Glei et al. 2007). A persistent but inefficient turning on or shutting off of adrenaline and other stress responses increases your risk for hypertension, coronary heart disease, and diabetes (McEwen 1998). The abuse of tobacco, high caffeine intake and amphetamines, and alcohol abuse to ameliorate stress does nothing to alleviate long-term stress and much to compromise your health.

You can reduce psychological stresses by developing and strengthening your ability to cope with real and imagined threats and adversity (Holden 1992). Indeed, developing and applying effective problem-solving and coping skills is a way to assert control. Actions to reduce stress and improve your health involve engaging in a healthy form of stress (Nelson and Cooper 2005). This propellant stress (p-stress) results from efforts to solve problems (Knaus 1994). But what do you target to solve?

The rest of this chapter concentrates on three main areas—liberating your mind, fortifying your body, and using your intellect, ingenuity, and will—to lighten your allostatic load, stabilize gains, and get ahead.

Liberating Your Mind

Liberate your mind from consistent errors, such as conning yourself into thinking that you can escape the consequences of procrastinating. Learning to recognize and end cognitive distortions and to build realistic evaluative skills is the cognitive way.

Rewrite the Script

The type of script you follow makes a big difference in how you live your life. For example, if you expect to live in a bubble of bliss, you are likely to feel exasperated.

What would Albert Ellis say of this? He'd suggest working at unconditional acceptance of yourself, of others, and of life. This boils down to taking things as they are, not as you wish or expect them to be.

Thirteenth century Dominican monk, theologian, and philosopher Thomas Aquinas is credited with saying, "Let me control what I can, accept what I can't, and know the difference between the two." In other words, you can't stop the ocean waves from pounding the shore, but you can still build sand castles or take a swim.

Use Your Mind Creatively and Constructively

Here are a few examples of how to build on the gains you've made in thinking clearly about your anxieties:

- Label any instance of distressing yourself over your distresses as a form of double trouble. Accurate labeling can make the process more understandable, controllable, and correctable. Reminding yourself that it's okay to be fallible can also help reduce the anxiety that is prompted by perfectionist thinking.

■ Practice a nonjudgmental view. Anxiety thinking has consequences; you can evaluate and debunk the thoughts to eliminate the consequences. Judging anxiety-evoking beliefs, without judging yourself, is a responsible action.

■ Look for incongruities in your thinking and act to resolve the incongruity. For example, if you label yourself a loser for backsliding, does that mean that everyone else is also a loser for having the same human tendency? If so, why? If not, why not? The chances are that you will see your original thought as an overgeneralization and possibly laugh when you do.

■ Construct a picture in your mind where you view yourself as steady on your feet when facing adversity. Under adverse conditions, imagine asking yourself, *What is the problem here that I can solve?* Imagine yourself solving the problem. Then do what you imagine.

■ Remind yourself that anxiety and fear thoughts are simply passing thoughts. They are part of how you are thinking at the moment. They neither last forever nor define the global you.

By drawing on your experiences and using your insight and practical judgment to clarify what is going on in and around you, you can continue to make positive changes.

Fortifying Your Body

Build your body to buffer the effects of multiple stresses. This is the biological way. To fortify your body against stress and disease, do not smoke, use illicit drugs, or drink excessively. Get regular dental care. Get a regular medical checkup. Exercise a minimum of thirty minutes a day. Get a good night's sleep. Eat sanely. This section takes a closer look at three of these areas: physical exercise, quality sleep, and eating sanely.

Physical Exercise

Although there is some evidence that exercise is helpful for reducing anxiety (Berk 2007), getting regular exercise is probably more of a general health initiative than it is a tool for reducing anxiety. Aerobic exercise helps to reduce your allostatic load, and as a by-product you may find that your heart rate and blood pressure will go down and your immune system will strengthen against disease. Even moderate exercise—walking four days a week for thirty minutes a session—can have a positive effect. Exercise also has short-term benefits. You are likely to feel better, pay better attention, and be able to concentrate better following physical exercise.

How you exercise is up to you. You have an obvious range of possibilities, from running in place, kayaking, riding a bike, working out at a gym, or walking on an inviting nature trail along a river, which can increase a sense of tranquility (see chapter 8). Activating music increases length of stride, vigor, and speed in synchronized walking (Leman et al. 2013). Consider transmitting this music through earphones as you walk.

Quality Sleep

Sleep loss is common among people with anxiety—perhaps as high as 70 percent (Belleville et al. 2010). Poorer sleep quality impairs your ability to regulate and reduce negative emotions (Mauss, Troy, and LeBourgeois 2013).

Without enough sleep, you may have problems concentrating on tasks and monitoring your anxiety-related thoughts and performances. Fatigue and being easily distracted can result in the pressure of running out of time on important tasks. Furthermore, worrying about getting things done can interfere with sleep. CBT delivers empirically supported methods for improving sleep patterns (Yang and Hsiao 2012).

Difficulty sleeping can result from such a wide range of causes that there is no one perfect system to relieve this state. Nevertheless, CBT techniques are especially useful for sleep problems related to worry and other stressful cognitions.

Say you feel stressed about work. It's midnight. You'd like to settle down and sleep. However, you lament yesterday's mistakes. You worry about tomorrow's problems. You are mindful of the sleep that you expect to lose. You don't want to feel fatigued tomorrow. You want to stop worrying so you can fall asleep. You tell yourself, *I have to stop worrying. I have to fall asleep.* Now you feel more awake than you did before. You want to stop fretting and free yourself from this emotional turmoil. You struggle to rid yourself of unwanted negative thoughts. You tell yourself, *I've got to fall asleep. I've got to fall asleep!* The harder you try, the more distress you feel.

Similarly if someone were to tell you not to think of a pink elephant, you would likely think of a pink elephant. To rid yourself of the pink elephant, you might try to distract yourself. You might think of a purple fox. Nevertheless, the pink elephant would remain on your mind. The harder you try to snuff out the image, the brighter it shines.

When you are emotionally charged, you are less likely to fall asleep. So how do you fall asleep? Start with a *passive volition* exercise, in which you practice an attitude of allowance. It boils down to this: *If I think of a pink elephant, I think of a pink elephant. So what?* By giving up the struggle, you may no longer have the pink elephant on your mind. Similarly, by allowing yourself to stay awake without trying not to, you might find that you are able to sleep after all.

Here are some other cognitive, emotive, and behavioral techniques for improving sleep patterns:

- Follow a regular sleep schedule. Go to bed when you are likely to feel sleepy.

- Recognize that even if you worry about staying awake, you will get rest of some kind if you lie still. You probably will slip into and out of sleep and get more rest than you think.

- Try white noise to muffle outside sounds. A good example of white noise would be the sound produced by a nonoperating television channel. Turn down the volume and put on the TV timer so that the set shuts off, say, in sixty minutes.

- Avoid associating your bed with wakefulness. When you are unable to sleep, get out of bed. Return in a few minutes. You may feel more ready to sleep.

- Do moderate aerobic exercise during the afternoon every day.

- Avoid ingesting coffee, cola, tea, chocolate, or other caffeine-containing substances seven hours before your regular bedtime.

- Avoid alcohol for three hours before going to bed. A glass of wine in the evening may cause you to feel relaxed, which may make it easier for you to fall asleep, but as the body breaks down alcohol, you compromise the quality of your sleep.

- Sleep in a well-ventilated room with a room temperature of sixty-five to sixty-eight degrees Fahrenheit. Sleep is associated with a drop in body temperature.

- Relax your body during periods of interrupted sleep. This has some restorative value. For example, squeeze and relax your main muscle groups. Imagine a fluffy cloud moving slowly across the sky.

- Plan to rise between 6:00 and 7:00 a.m. Sleeping late increases the risk of depression.

- Give yourself something to compete with negative cognitions. Count backward from one thousand by threes. Think of a positive event for each negative thought.

- If you routinely have trouble sleeping because you anxiously reflect on the trials and tribulations of the preceding day, adopt a coping perspective. Whenever feasible and reasonable, resolve daily conflicts as they arise.

If you know or suspect that you have a medical condition affecting your sleep, make a medical appointment.

Eating Sanely

Active efforts to exercise and maintain a healthy weight reduce cardiac risk up to 79 percent (Völler 2006). When you are overweight, weight loss appears to improve health across the board (Foreyt 2005). There is an obesity paradox worth noting: you can have a normal weight but carry excess fat, and this increases your risk for coronary heart disease (Chaikriangkrai et al. 2014).

There is currently no definitive study on whether being overweight causes anxiety (self-consciousness about body image) or whether anxiety causes you to be overweight (using food for comfort). The key word, however, is "sometimes." Sometimes it is one way, sometimes another.

Whether excess fat is a result of anxiety or a cause, the extra stress on the body is an allostatic load factor.

Habits of eating excessively or inadequately do not easily yield to the intellectual decision to adopt sane eating habits. This is especially the case when anxious and you use food for comfort, or when you starve yourself because you are anxious over your appearance and obsessed with losing weight.

Setting weight goals that you need to stretch to achieve may be a wiser course of action than setting them too low (De Vet et al. 2013). However, it's the process of how you go about making and sustaining healthy eating changes that makes the difference. The no-diet-diet plan is an example of a process goal that you can stretch to achieve (Knaus 2012). With this plan, you attend to both the process—how you go about fortifying yourself by eating sanely—and the outcome of minimizing excess fat. Use it to shed fat if you carry too much or to put on weight if you are too lean:

- Set a desirable weight—something you can stretch for but also achieve.

- Plan to consume daily the number of calories you need to reach and maintain your desired weight.

- Eat appealing food in proper proportions with the necessary nutrients for a balanced diet.

Suppose you are a five-foot-five forty-year-old woman who weighs 150 pounds, and you want to weigh 125 pounds to prevent future health problems associated with carrying too much fat. You exercise moderately.

With moderate exercise, it takes about 2,100 calories a day to maintain your weight at 150 pounds. If you want to weigh and stay at 125 pounds, it would take about 1,919 calories per day. There are many free calorie calculators on the Internet to figure out your daily calorie requirements to reach and maintain your desired weight given your activity level. Some calculators will give you a time frame for how long it will take to reach your goal. As a rule of thumb, you lose a pound for each 3,600 fewer calories you consume or burn off by exercising. You gain a pound for every 3,600 extra calories you consume.

If you are like most people, you won't establish perfect control over the no-diet process. Expect variability in both the process and the result, and you won't be disappointed. Adjustments are typically necessary. If you have an illness, you may not be able to moderately exercise. Don't look for perfection; rather, work at improving the process. By the time you reach your desired weight, you will have developed eating habits that are commensurate with that weight.

It would be challenging to measure every food item for its caloric value and then to count them up each day. Instead, educate yourself on foods that are calorie rich and those that have greater nutritional value without the extra calories. You might try a substitution technique in which you replace a fattening food with a more nutritious and lower calorie food. For example, if you pack on fat by consuming a calorie-rich brownie a day, replace it with a healthier alternative, such as a square of dark chocolate.

Note that you needn't give up chocolate. In fact, cocoa has been shown to have a calming effect on nonanxious folk, and the next wave of research will be to see whether cocoa polyphenols can have a calming effect on folks with higher levels of anxieties (Pase et al. 2013). In a small-scale study, nursing students who consumed fifty grams of dark chocolate a day reported reductions in anxiety and depression within three days (Lua and Wong 2011).

Building Positive Lifestyle Patterns

A basic theme throughout this book is how to use cognitive, emotional tolerance, and behavioral methods to overcome parasitic anxieties and fears. Intellect, ingenuity, and will overlay this process. Using these six complementary processes, you can establish a plan to prevent your anxieties and fears from coming back. Reducing these negatives is positive. Here's an example:

A Preventive Maintenance Plan

Prevention Factor	Intellect	Ingenuity	Will
Cognitive	Recognize anxiety-and-fear thinking when it first starts to kindle.	Maintain a healthy perspective by recognizing and questioning incongruities. Be alert for double-trouble reasoning. Look for new ways to address incongruities.	Will is not something you can dial up, but you can create conditions for strengthening it. Focus on your prime incentives for preventing anxieties and fears from coming back. How much do those incentives matter?
Emotional tolerance	Identify discomfort-dodging urges that accompany anxiety thinking. If you have an urge to retreat, can you think of a better way to manage your thinking?	Look for adaptive ways to accept the discomfort. Create a positive coping image of yourself managing the problem signaled by the discomfort. Then build in accepting discomfort as part of your plan to translate the coping image into action.	The will to avoid discomfort can be strong. What other emotions can you mobilize to live through discomfort, so that you no longer fear it? Is it possible for you to pit forcefulness against a will to retreat? Can you imagine yourself squarely facing the fear?

| Behavioral | Determine what behaviors extend from anxiety thinking and sensations. What actions can you take to counter them? For example, rather than retreat out of fear of defeat, respond assertively by moving to conquer the fear. | Taking creative actions can strengthen secondary prevention. Can you write a poem extolling the benefits of prevention that can guide you on this path? Can you give a creative flair to a to-do list of preventive maintenance techniques? | Consider the benefits you get from asserting your will to review and renew behavioral techniques to stop anxiety-and-fear reactions from coming back. Keep them firmly in mind. |

EXERCISE: YOUR PREVENTIVE MAINTENANCE PLAN

Design your own preventive maintenance plan, specifying the cognitive, emotional tolerance, and behavioral methods that you will use, along with your intellect, ingenuity, and will, to keep your anxieties and fears at bay. Then put your plan into practice.

Your Cognitive-Emotive-Behavioral Preventive Maintenance Plan

Prevention Factor	Intellect	Ingenuity	Will
Cognitive			
Emotional tolerance			
Behavioral			

There are two natural areas that most people can benefit from addressing. The first is to reduce the negatives in your life. The second is to stretch for positive experiences that are in your enlightened interest. Once you've progressed in these two directions, continue with your preventative maintenance plan.

Top Tip: Deal with Anxiety Early

Psychologist Nancy Knaus, PhD, MBA, and coauthor of *Fearless Job Hunting*, shares her top tip on anxiety prevention:

"If you feel a needless anxiety stirring about something in your life, take preventative steps to stop anxiety from getting a foothold:

1. Keep perspective on what is most important in your life. It can be family. It can be a passionate pursuit. Emphasize what you value over what you fear.

2. Separate yourself from your anxiety symptoms. You are not an anxious person. You are a person who sometimes experiences anxiety and who wants to experience this feeling less often. By not identifying with your anxiety, you are freer to release it.

3. Go on the offensive. Take the most basic step that you can take to advance against the anxiety you experience. If you have trouble motivating yourself to take this step first, remind yourself that you act against anxiety to prevent anxiety from interfering with what you value most in life."

Self-improvement comes down to this: Stay focused on the big-picture prize, the enjoyment of your life. Maintain a self-observant perspective. Stretch to see how far you can advance your enlightened interests. Look for opportunities where you can contribute to the welfare of others. Through this process, you will do more than emotionally survive; you'll thrive.

YOUR PROGRESS REPORT

Write down what you learned from this chapter and what actions you plan to take. Then record what resulted from taking these actions and what you've gained.

What are three key ideas that you took away from this chapter?

1.

2.

3.

What top three actions can you take to combat a specific anxiety or fear?

1.

2.

3.

What resulted when you took these actions?

1.

2.

3.

What did you gain from taking action? What would you do differently next time?

1.

2.

3.

Suggested Reading

Anger Management: The Complete Treatment Guidebook for Practitioners (The Practical Therapist Series), by Howard Kassinove and Raymond Chip Tafrate. Atascadero, CA: Impact Publishers, 2002.

The Beck Diet Solution Weight Loss Workbook: The Six-Week Plan to Train Your Brain to Think Like a Thin Person, by Judith S. Beck. Birmingham, AL: Oxmoor House, 2007.

Changeology: Five Steps to Realizing Your Goals and Resolutions, by John Norcross, Kristin Loberg, and Jonathon Norcross. New York: Simon and Schuster, 2012.

The Cognitive Behavioral Workbook for Depression, second edition, by William Knaus. Oakland, CA: New Harbinger Publications, 2012.

The Dutiful Worrier: How to Stop Compulsive Worry Without Feeling Guilty, by Elliot D. Cohen. Oakland, CA: New Harbinger Publications, 2011.

Fearless Job Hunting: Powerful Psychological Strategies for Getting the Job You Want, by William Knaus, Samuel Klarreich, Russell Grieger, and Nancy Knaus. Oakland, CA: New Harbinger Publications, 2010.

Get Out of Your Mind and Into Your Life, by Steven C. Hayes, with Spencer Smith. Oakland, CA: New Harbinger Publications, 2005.

A Guide to Shameless Happiness, by Will Ross. Amazon Digital Services, Inc., 2012.

Healing, Volume 2: Reflections for Clergy, Chaplains and Counselors, by George Morelli. Fairfax, VA: Eastern Christian Publications, 2012.

Homer the Homely Hound Dog, by Edward Garcia and Nina Pellegrini. New York: Institute for Rational Emotive Therapy, 1974.

Pressure Proofing: How to Increase Personal Effectiveness on the Job and Anywhere Else for That Matter, by Samuel Klarreich. New York: Routledge, 2007.

The Procrastination Workbook, by William Knaus. Oakland, CA: New Harbinger Publications, 2002.

Rational-Emotive and Cognitive-Behavior Therapy, vol. 10, no. 1, edited by Russell Grieger and Paul Woods. New York: Human Sciences Press, 1992.

Rational and Irrational Beliefs: Research, Theory, and Clinical Practice, edited by Daniel David, Steven Lynn, and Albert Ellis. New York: Oxford University Press, 2009.

The REBT Super-Activity Guide: 52 Weeks of REBT for Clients, Groups, Students, and YOU!, by Pamela D. Garcy. CreateSpace: Independent Publishing Platform, 2009.

Saving My Life: A Least Likely to Succeed Success Story, by Joel Block. Amazon Digital Services, Inc. 2011.

The Search for Fulfillment: Revolutionary New Research That Reveals the Secret to Long-term Happiness, by Susan Krauss Whitbourne. New York: Ballantine Books, 2010.

The 60-Second Shrink: 101 Strategies for Staying Sane in a Crazy World, by Arnold A. Lazarus and Clifford N. Lazarus. San Luis Obispo, CA: Impact Publishers, 1997.

Your Perfect Right: Assertiveness and Equality in Your Life and Relationships, 9th edition, by Robert Alberti and Michael Emmons. Atascadero, CA: Impact Publishers, 2008.

References

Abraham, A. 2013. "The World According to Me: Personal Relevance and the Medial Prefrontal Cortex." *Frontiers in Human Neuroscience* 7: 341. doi: 10.3389/fnhum.2013.00341.

Adler, A. 1927. *Understanding Human Nature.* New York: Garden City Publishing.

Ainslie, G. 2005. "Précis of *Breakdown of Will*." *Behavioral and Brain Sciences* 28 (5): 635–50.

Alberti, R., and M. Emmons. 2008. *Your Perfect Right: Assertiveness and Equality in Your Life and Relationships.* 9th ed. Atascadero, CA: Impact Publishers.

Allen, L. B., K. S. White, D. H. Barlow, M. K. Shear, J. M. Gorman, and S. W. Woods. 2010. "Cognitive-Behavior Therapy (CBT) for Panic Disorder: Relationship of Anxiety and Depression Comorbidity with Treatment Outcome." *Journal of Psychopathology and Behavioral Assessment* 32 (2): 185–92.

Allport, G. W., and H. S. Odbert. 1936. *Trait-Names: A Psycho-Lexical Study.* Albany, NY: Psychological Review Company.

Arnold, M. B. 1960. *Emotion and Personality.* New York: Columbia University Press.

Ashbaugh, A., M. M. Antony, A. Liss, L. J. Summerfeldt, R. E. McCabe, and R. P. Swinson. 2007. "Changes in Perfectionism Following Cognitive-Behavioral Treatment for Social Phobia." *Depression and Anxiety* 24 (3): 169–77.

Åsli, O., and M. A. Flaten. 2012. "How Fast Is Fear? Automatic and Controlled Processing in Conditioned Fear." *Journal of Psychophysiology* 26 (1): 20–28.

Averina, M., O. Nilssen, T. Brenn, J. Brox, V. L. Arkhipovsky, and A. G. Kalinin. 2005. "Social and Lifestyle Determinants of Depression, Anxiety, Sleeping Disorders and Self-Evaluated Quality of Life in Russia: A Population-Based Study in Arkhangelsk." *Social Psychiatry and Psychiatric Epidemiology* 40 (7): 511–18.

Baillie, A., and C. Sannibale. 2007. "Anxiety and Drug and Alcohol Problems." In *Clinical Handbook of Co-Existing Mental Health and Drug and Alcohol Problems*, edited by A. Baker and R. Velleman. New York: Routledge/Taylor and Francis Group.

Bandura, A. 1988. "Self-Efficacy Conception of Anxiety." *Anxiety Research* 1(2): 77–98.

———. 1997. *Self-Efficacy: The Exercise of Control*. New York: W.H. Freeman and Company.

———. 1999. "Self-Efficacy: Toward a Unifying Theory of Behavioral Change." In *The Self in Social Psychology*, edited by R. F. Baumeister. New York: Psychology Press.

Bar-Haim, Y., D. Lamy, L. Pergamin, M. J. Bakermans-Kranenburg, and M. H. van Ijzendoorn. 2007. "Threat-Related Attentional Bias in Anxious and Nonanxious Individuals: A Meta-Analytic Study." *Psychological Bulletin* 133 (1): 1–24.

Barlow, D. H. 1988. *Anxiety and Its Disorders*. New York: Guilford Press.

Barrett, L. F., E. Bliss-Moreau, S. L. Duncan, S. L. Rauch, and C. I. Wright. 2007. "The Amygdala and the Experience of Affect." *Social, Cognitive, and Affective Neuroscience* 2 (2): 73–83.

Barton J., M. Griffin, and J. Pretty. 2012. "Exercise-, Nature- and Socially Interactive-Based Initiatives Improve Mood and Self-Esteem in the Clinical Population." *Perspectives in Public Health* 132 (2): 89–96.

Barton J., and J. Pretty. 2010. "What Is the Best Dose of Nature and Green Exercise for Improving Mental Health? A Multi-Study Analysis." *Environmental Science and Technology* 44 (10): 3947–55.

Bateson, M., B. Brilot, and D. Nettle. 2011. "Anxiety: An Evolutionary Approach." *Canadian Journal of Psychiatry* 56 (12): 707–15.

Baumeister, H., and M. Härter. 2007. "Prevalence of Mental Disorders Based on General Population Surveys." *Social Psychiatry and Psychiatric Epidemiology* 42 (7): 537–46.

Beck, A. T., and D. J. Dozois. 2011, "Cognitive Therapy: Current Status and Future Directions." *Annual Review of Medicine* 62: 397–409.

Beesdo, K., A. Bittner, D. S. Pine, M. B. Stein, M. Hofler, R. Lieb and H.-S. Wittchen. 2007. "Incidence of Social Anxiety Disorder and the Consistent Risk for Secondary Depression In the First Three Decades of Life." *Archives of General Psychiatry* 64 (8): 903-912.

Belleville, G., H. Cousineau, K. Levrier, M. E. St-Pierre-Delorme, and A. Marchand. 2010. "The Impact of Cognitive-Behavior Therapy for Anxiety Disorders on Concomitant Sleep Disturbances: A Meta-Analysis." *Journal of Anxiety Disorders* 24 (4): 379–86.

Benight, C. C., and A. Bandura. 2004. "Social Cognitive Theory of Posttraumatic Recovery: The Role of Perceived Self-Efficacy." *Behaviour Research and Therapy* 42 (10): 1129–48.

Berk, M. 2007. "Should We Be Targeting Exercise as a Routine Mental Health Intervention?" *Acta Neuropsychiatrica* 19 (3): 217–18.

Berkowitz, R. L., J. D. Coplan, D. P. Reddy, and J. M. Gorman. 2007. "The Human Dimension: How the Prefrontal Cortex Modulates the Subcortical Fear Response." *Reviews in the Neurosciences* 18 (3-4): 191–208.

Berman, M. G., J. Jonides, and S. Kaplan. 2008. "The Cognitive Benefits of Interacting with Nature." *Psychological Science* 19 (12): 1207–212.

Birrella, J., K. Meares, A. Wilkinson, and M. Freeston. 2011. "Toward a Definition of Intolerance of Uncertainty: A Review of Factor Analytical Studies of the Intolerance of Uncertainty Scale." *Clinical Psychology Review* 31 (7): 1198–208.

Bishop, S. R. 2007. "What We Really Know About Mindfulness-Based Stress Reduction." In vol. 2 of *The Praeger Handbook on Stress and Coping*, edited by A. Monat, R. S. Lazarus, and G. Reevy. Westport, CT: Praeger Publishers.

Blascovich, J., E. Vanman, W. B. Mendes, and S. Dickerson. 2011. *Social Psychophysiology for Social and Personality Psychology*. New York: Sage.

Boswell, J. F., T. J. Farchione, S. Sauer-Zavala, H. W. Murray, M. R. Fortune, and D. H. Barlow. 2013. "Anxiety Sensitivity and Interoceptive Exposure: A Transdiagnostic Construct and Change Strategy." *Behavior Therapy* 44 (3): 417-431.

Brown, D. K., J. L. Barton, and V. F. Gladwell. 2013. "Viewing Nature Scenes Positively Affects Recovery of Autonomic Function Following Acute-Mental Stress." *Environmental Science and Technology* 47 (11): 5562–69.

Buhr, K., and M. J. Dugas. 2006. "Investigating the Construct Validity of Intolerance of Uncertainty and Its Unique Relationship with Worry." *Journal of Anxiety Disorders* 20 (2): 222–36.

Butler, A. C., J. E. Chapman, E. M. Forman, and A. T. Beck. 2006. "The Empirical Status of Cognitive-Behavioral Therapy: A Review of Meta-Analyses." *Clinical Psychology Review* 26 (1): 17–31.

Butler, D. L., J. B. Mattingley, R. Cunnington, and T. Suddendorf. 2013. "Different Neural Processes Accompany Self-Recognition in Photographs Across the Lifespan: An ERP Study Using Dizygotic Twins." *PLoS One* 8 (9): e72586. doi:10.1371/journal.pone.0072586. Collection 2013.

Bystritsky, A., L. Kerwin, N. Niv, J. L. Natoli, N. Abrahami, R. Klap, K. Wells, and A. S. Young. 2010. "Clinical and Subthreshold Panic Disorder." *Depression and Anxiety* 27 (4): 381–89.

Cammin-Nowak, S., S. Helbig-Lang, T. Lang, A. T. Gloster, L. Fehm, A. L. Gerlach, et al. 2013. "Specificity of Homework Compliance Effects on Treatment Outcome in CBT: Evidence from a Controlled Trial on Panic Disorder and Agoraphobia." *Journal of Clinical Psychology* 69 (6): 616–29.

Campbell-Sills, L., C. D. Sherbourne, P. Roy-Byrne, M. G. Craske, G. Sullivan, A. Bystritsky, et al. 2012. "Effects of Co-occurring Depression on Treatment for Anxiety Disorders: Analysis of

Outcomes from a Large Primary Care Effectiveness Trial." *The Journal of Clinical Psychiatry* 73 (12): 1509–16.

Carlson, J., R. E. Watts, and M. Maniacci. 2006. *Adlerian Therapy: Theory and Practice.* Washington, DC: American Psychological Association.

Chaikriangkrai, K., M. Kassi, S. K. Bala, F. Nabi, and S. M. Chang. 2014. "Atherosclerosis Burden in Patients with Acute Chest Pain: Obesity Paradox." *ISRN Obesity* 2014: 634717. http://dx.doi.org/10.1155/2014/634717.

Clara, I. P., B. J. Cox, and M. W. Enns. 2007. "Assessing Self-Critical Perfectionism in Clinical Depression." *Journal of Personality Assessment* 88 (3): 309–16.

Clauss, J. A., and J. U. Blackford. 2012. "Behavioral Inhibition and Risk for Developing Social Anxiety Disorder: A Meta-Analytic Study." *Journal of the American Academy of Child and Adolescent Psychiatry* 51 (10): 1066–75.

Cody, M. W., and B. A. Teachman. 2011. "Global and Local Evaluations of Public Speaking Performance in Social Anxiety." *Behavior Therapy* 42 (4): 601–11.

Collerton, D. 2013. "Psychotherapy and Brain Plasticity." *Frontiers in Psychology* 4: 548. http://www.ncbi.nlm.nih.gov/pmc/articles/PMC3764373/

Cooley, C. H. 1902. *Human Nature and the Social Order.* New York: Charles Scribner's Sons.

Craig, A. 2009. "How Do You Feel—Now? The Anterior Insula and Human Awareness." *Nature Reviews: Neuroscience* 101: 59–70.

Craske, M. G. 2012. "Transdiagnostic Treatment for Anxiety and Depression." *Depression and Anxiety* 29 (9): 749–53.

Crome, E., A. Baillie, and A. Taylor. 2012. "Are Male and Female Responses to Social Phobia Diagnostic Criteria Comparable?" *International Journal of Methods in Psychiatric Research* 21 (3): 222–31.

Cuijpers, P., M. Sijbrandij, S. Koole, M. Huibers, M. Berking, and G. Andersson. 2014. "Psychological Treatment of Generalized Anxiety Disorder: A Meta-Analysis." *Clinical Psychology Review* 34 (2): 130–40.

Das, A. 2013. "Anxiety Disorders in Bipolar I Mania: Prevalence, Effect on Illness Severity, and Treatment Implications." *Indian Journal of Psychological Medicine* 35 (1): 53–59.

Davey, G. C. L., F. Eldridge, J. Drost, and B. A. MacDonald. 2007. "What Ends a Worry Bout? An Analysis of Changes in Mood and Stop Rule Use Across the Catastrophising Interview Task." *Behaviour Research and Therapy* 45 (6): 1231-43.

Davis, M. 1998. "Are Different Parts of the Extended Amygdala Involved in Fear Versus Anxiety?" *Biological Psychiatry* 44 (12): 1239–47.

De Vet, E., R. M. Nelissen, M. Zeelenberg and D. T. De Ridder, 2013. "Ain't No Mountain High Enough? Setting High Weight Loss Goals Predict Effort and Short-Term Weight Loss." *Journal of Health Psychology* 18 (5): 638–47.

Debiec, J., and J. E. LeDoux. 2009. "The Amygdala and the Neural Pathways of Fear." In *Post-Traumatic Stress Disorder: Basic Science and Clinical Practice*, edited by P. J. Shiromani, T. M. Keane, and J. E. LeDoux. Totowa, NJ: Humana Press.

Dollard, J. 1942. *Victory Over Fear*. New York: Reynal and Hitchcock.

Dugas, M. J., P. Savard, A. Gaudet, J. Turcotte, N. Laugesen, M. Robichaud, K. Francis, and N. Koerner. 2007. "Can the Components of a Cognitive Model Predict the Severity of Generalized Anxiety Disorder?" *Behavior Therapy* 38 (2): 169–78.

Dunn, M. C. 1976. "Landscape with Photographs: Testing the Preference Approach to Landscape Evaluation." *Journal of Environmental Management* 4: 15–26.

Dutton, D. 2003. "Aesthetics and Evolutionary Psychology." In *The Oxford Handbook for Aesthetics*, edited by J. Levinson. New York: Oxford University Press.

Eberth, J., and P. Sedlmeier. 2012. "The Effects of Mindfulness Meditation: A Meta-Analysis." *Mindfulness* 3 (3): 174–89.

Egan, S. J., J. P. Piek, M. J. Dyck, and C. S. Rees. 2007. "The Role of Dichotomous Thinking and Rigidity in Perfectionism." *Behaviour Research and Therapy* 45 (8): 1813–22.

Egan, S. J., T. D. Wade, and R. Shafran. 2011. "Perfectionism As a Transdiagnostic Process: A Clinical Review." *Clinical Psychology Review* 31 (2): 203–12.

Ellis, A. 2000. *How to Control Your Anxiety Before It Controls You*. New York: Citadel Press.

———. 2008. "Rational Emotive Behavior Therapy." In *The Quick Theory Reference Guide: A Resource for Expert and Novice Mental Health Professionals*, edited by K. Jordan. Hauppauge, NY: Nova Science Publishers.

Ellis, A., and R. A. Harper. 1997. *A Guide to Rational Living*. 3rd ed. North Hollywood, CA: Wilshire Book Company.

Emerson, R. W. 1870. *Society and Solitude*. Cambridge MA: University Press: Welch Bigelow and Co.

Engels, A. S., W. Heller, A. Mohanty, J. D. Herrington, M. T. Banich, A. G. Webb, and G. A. Miller. 2007. "Specificity of Regional Brain Activity in Anxiety Types During Emotion Processing." *Psychophysiology* 44 (3): 352–63.

Epictetus. 2004. *Discourses* (Books 1 and 2). NY: Dover Publications.

Eppley, K. R., A. I. Abrams, and J. Shear. 1989. "Differential Effects of Relaxation Techniques on Trait Anxiety: A Meta-Analysis." *Journal of Clinical Psychology* 45 (6): 957–74.

Evans, S., S. Ferrando, M. Findler, C. Stowell, C. Smart, and D. Haglin. 2008. "Mindfulness-Based Cognitive Therapy for Generalized Anxiety Disorder." *Journal of Anxiety Disorders* 22 (4): 716–21.

Fairburn, C. G., Z. Cooper, H. A. Doll, M. E. O'Connor, K. Bohn, D. M. Hawker, J. A. Wales, and R. L. Palmer. 2009. "Transdiagnostic Cognitive-Behavioral Therapy for Patients with Eating Disorders: A Two-Site Trial with Sixty-Week Follow-Up." *The American Journal of Psychiatry* 166 (3): 311–19.

Falk, J. H., and J. D. Balling. 2010. "Evolutionary Influence on Human Landscape Preference." *Environment and Behavior* 42 (4): 479–93.

Feltz, D. L. 1982. "Path Analysis of the Causal Elements in Bandura's Theory of Self-Efficacy and an Anxiety-Based Model of Avoidance Behavior." *Journal of Personality and Social Psychology* 42 (4): 764–81.

Fergus, T. A., D. P. Valentiner, P. B. McGrath, S. Gier-Lonsway, and S. Jencius. 2013. "The Cognitive Attentional Syndrome: Examining Relations with Mood and Anxiety Symptoms and Distinctiveness from Psychological Inflexibility in a Clinical Sample." *Psychiatry Research* 210 (1): 215–19.

Foreyt, J. P. 2005. "Need for Lifestyle Intervention: How to Begin." *American Journal of Cardiology* 96 (4A): 11E–14E.

Furukawa, T. A., Y. Nakano, T. Funayama, S. Ogawa, T. Ietsugu, Y. Noda, J. Chen, N. Watanabe, and T. Akechi. 2013. "Cognitive-Behavioral Therapy Modifies the Naturalistic Course of Social Anxiety Disorder: Findings from an ABA Design Study in Routine Clinical Practices." *Psychiatry and Clinical Neurosciences* 67 (3): 139–47.

Gadermann, A. M., J. Alonso, G. Vilagut, A. M. Zaslavsky, and R. C. Kessler. 2012. "Co-Morbidity and Disease Burden in the National Comorbidity Survey Replication (NCS-R)." *Depression and Anxiety* 29 (9): 797–806.

Galante, J., S. J. Iribarren, and P. F. Pearce. 2013. "Effects of Mindfulness-Based Cognitive Therapy on Mental Disorders: A Systematic Review and Meta-Analysis of Randomised Controlled Trials." *Journal of Research in Nursing* 18 (2): 133–55.

Gallagher, M. W., K. Naragon-Gainey, and T. A. Brown. 2014. "Perceived Control Is a Transdiagnostic Predictor of Cognitive-Behavior Therapy Outcome for Anxiety Disorders." *Cognitive Therapy and Research* 38 (1): 10–22.

Gallagher, M. W., L. A. Payne, K. S. White, K. M. Shear, S. W. Woods, J. M. Gorman, and D. H. Barlow. 2013. "Mechanisms of Change in Cognitive Behavioral Therapy for Panic Disorder: The Unique Effects of Self-Efficacy and Anxiety Sensitivity." *Behaviour Research and Therapy* 51 (11): 767–77.

Galvao-de Almeida, A., G. M. de Araujo Filho, A. A. Berberian, C. Trezsniak, F. Nery-Fernandes, C. A. Araujo Neto, A. P. Jackowski, A. Miranda-Scippa, and I. R. de Oliveira. 2013. "The

Impacts of Cognitive-Behavioral Therapy on the Treatment of Phobic Disorders Measured by Functional Neuroimaging Techniques: A Systematic Review." *Revista Brasileira de Psiquiatria* 35 (3): 279–83. (English translation).

Glei, D. A., N. Goldman, Y. Chuang, and M. Weinstein. 2007. "Do Chronic Stressors Lead to Physiological Disregulation? Testing the Theory of Allostatic Load." *Psychosomatic Medicine* 69 (8): 769–76.

Gloster, A. T., C. Hauke, M. Höfler, F. Einsle, T. Fydrich, A. Hamm, A. Sthröhle, and H. U. Wittchen. 2013. "Long-Term Stability of Cognitive Behavioral Therapy Effects for Panic Disorder with Agoraphobia: A Two-Year Follow-Up Study." *Behaviour Research and Therapy* 51 (12): 830–39.

Goldapple, K., Z. Segal, C. Garson, M. Lau, P. Bieling, S. Kennedy, and H. Mayberg. 2004. "Modulation of Cortical-Limbic Pathways in Major Depression: Treatment-Specific Effects of Cognitive Behavior Therapy." *Archives of General Psychiatry* 61 (1): 34–41.

Golkar, A., M. Bellander, and A. Öhman. 2013. "Temporal Properties of Fear Extinction—Does Time Matter?" *Behavioral Neuroscience* 127 (1): 59–69.

Goossens, L., S. Sunaert, R. Peeters, E. J. Griez, and K. R. Schruers. 2007. "Amygdala Hyperfunction in Phobic Fear Normalizes After Exposure." *Biological Psychiatry* 62 (10): 1119–25.

Gorwood, P. 2004. "Generalized Anxiety Disorder and Major Depressive Disorder Comorbidity: An Example of Genetic Pleiotropy?" *European Psychiatry* 19 (1): 27–33.

Green, S. M., M. M. Antony, R. E. McCabe, and M. A. Watling. 2007. "Frequency of Fainting, Vomiting and Incontinence in Panic Disorder: A Descriptive Study." *Clinical Psychology and Psychotherapy* 14 (3): 189–97.

Gregory, R. J., S. S. Canning, T. W. Lee, and J. C. Wise. 2004. "Cognitive Bibliotherapy for Depression: A Meta-Analysis." *Professional Psychology: Research and Practice* 35 (3): 275–80.

Ham, T. E., V. Bonnelle, P. Hellyer, S. Jilka, I. H. Robertson, R. Leech, and D. J. Sharp. 2014. "The Neural Basis of Impaired Self-Awareness After Traumatic Brain Injury." *Brain* 137 (2): 586–97.

Hazlett-Stevens, H., and M. G. Craske. 2008. "Breathing Retraining and Diaphragmatic Breathing Techniques." In *Cognitive Behavior Therapy: Applying Empirically Supported Techniques in Your Practice*, edited by W. T. O'Donohue and J. E. Fisher. 2nd ed. Hoboken, NJ: John Wiley and Sons.

Hirai, M., and G. A. Clum. 2006. "A Meta-Analytic Study of Self-Help Interventions for Anxiety Problems." *Behavior Therapy* 37 (2): 99–111.

Hofmann, S., A. Asnaani, I. J. J. Vonk, A. T. Sawyer, and A. Fang. 2012. "The Efficacy of Cognitive Behavioral Therapy: A Review of Meta-analyses." *Cognitive Therapy and Research* 36 (5): 427–440.

Holden, G. 1992. "The Relationship of Self-Efficacy Appraisals to Subsequent Health Related Outcomes: A Meta-Analysis." *Social Work in Health Care* 16 (1): 53–93.

Holle, C., and R. Ingram. 2008. "On the Psychological Hazards of Self-Criticism." In *Self-Criticism and Self-Enhancement: Theory, Research, and Clinical Implications*, edited by E. C. Chang. Washington, DC: American Psychological Association.

Hölzel, B. K., J. Carmody, M. Vangel, C. Congleton, S. M. Yerramsetti, T. Gard, and S. W. Lazar. 2011. "Mindfulness Practice Leads to Increases in Regional Brain Gray Matter Density." *Psychiatry Research: Neuroimaging* 191 (1): 36–43.

Indovina, I., T. W. Robbins, A. O. Núñez-Elizalde, B. D. Dunn, and S. J. Bishop. 2011. "Fear-Conditioning Mechanisms Associated with Trait Vulnerability to Anxiety in Humans." *Neuron* 69 (3): 563–71.

Ingram, R. E., W. Ramel, D. Chavira, and C. Scher. 2005. "Social Anxiety and Depression." In *The Essential Handbook of Social Anxiety for Clinicians*, edited by W. R. Crozier and L. E. Alden. New York: John Wiley and Sons.

Jebb, R. C. 1909. *The Rhetoric of Aristotle*. United Kingdom: Cambridge University Press.

Kabat-Zinn, J. 1990. *Full Catastrophe Living*. New York: Delta Publishing.

———. 2003. "Mindfulness-Based Interventions in Context: Past, Present, and Future." *Clinical Psychology: Science and Practice* 10 (2): 144–56.

Katerndahl, D. A., and J. P. Realini. 1993. "Lifetime Prevalence of Panic States." *The American Journal of Psychiatry* 150 (2): 246–49.

Kelly, G. 1955. *The Psychology of Personal Constructs*. New York: Norton.

Kertz, S. J., J. S. Bigda-Peyton, D. H. Rosmarin, and T. Björgvinsson. 2012. "The Importance of Worry Across Diagnostic Presentations: Prevalence, Severity and Associated Symptoms in a Partial Hospital Setting." *Journal of Anxiety Disorders* 26 (1): 126–33.

Kessler, R. C., S. Avenevoli, E. J. Costello, K. Georgiades, J. G. Green, M. J. Gruber, J. P. He, D. Koretz, K. A. McLaughlin, M. Petukhova, N. A. Sampson, A. M. Zaslavsky and K. R. Merikangas. 2012. "Prevalence, Persistence, and Sociodemographic Correlates of DSM-IV Disorders in the National Comorbidity Survey Replication Adolescent Supplement." *Archives of General Psychiatry* 69 (4): 372–80.

Kessler, R. C., P. Berglund, O. Demler, R. Jin, K. R. Merikangas, and E. E. Walters. 2005. "Lifetime Prevalence and Age-of-Onset Distributions of DSM-IV Disorders in the National Comorbidity Survey Replication." *Archives of General Psychiatry* 62 (6): 593–602.

Kessler, R. C., B. J. Cox, J. G. Green, J. Ormel, K. A. McLaughlin, K. R. Merikangas, et al. 2011. "The Effects of Latent Variables in the Development of Comorbidity Among Common Mental Disorders." *Depression and Anxiety* 28 (1): 29–39.

Kessler, R. C., M. Petukhova, N. A. Sampson, A. M. Zaslavsky, and H. U. Wittchen. 2012. "Twelve-Month and Lifetime Prevalence and Lifetime Morbid Risk of Anxiety and Mood Disorders in the United States." *International Journal of Methods in Psychiatric Research* 21 (3): 169–84.

Khoury, B., T. Lecomte, G. Fortin, M. Masse, P. Therien, V. Bouchard, M. A. Chapleau, K. Paquin, and S. G. Hofmann. 2013. "Mindfulness-Based Therapy: A Comprehensive Meta-Analysis." *Clinical Psychology Review* 33 (6): 763–7

Kircher, T., V. Arolt, A. Jansen, M. Pyka, I. Reinhardt, T. Kellermann et al. 2013. "Effect of Cognitive-Behavioral Therapy on Neural Correlates of Fear Conditioning in Panic Disorder." *Biological Psychiatry* 73 (1): 93–101.

Knaus, W. 1982. *How to Get Out of a Rut.* Englewood Cliffs, NJ: Prentice-Hall.

———. 1994. *Change Your Life Now.* New York: John Wiley and Sons.

———. 2000. *Take Charge Now.* New York: John Wiley and Sons.

———. 2012. *The Cognitive Behavioral Workbook for Depression.* 2nd ed. Oakland, CA: New Harbinger Publications.

Kobayakawa, K., R. Kobayakawa, H. Matsumoto, Y. Oka, T. Imai, M Ikawa et al. 2007. "Innate Versus Learned Odour Processing in the Mouse Olfactory Bulb." *Nature* 450 (7169): 503–8.

Krause, L., P. G. Enticott, A. Zangen, and P. B. Fitzgerald. 2012. "The Role of Medial Prefrontal Cortex in Theory of Mind: A Deep rTMS Study." *Behavioural Brain Research* 228 (1): 87–90.

Kravitz, D. J., C. S. Peng, and C. I. Baker. 2011. "Real-World Scene Representations in High-Level Visual Cortex: It's the Spaces More Than the Places." *Journal of Neuroscience* 31 (20): 7322–33.

Kuo, F. E. 2001. "Coping with Poverty: Impacts of Environment and Attention in the Inner City." *Environment and Behavior* 33 (1): 5–34.

Kweon, B. S., R. S. Ulrich, V. D. Walker, and L. G. Tassinary. 2008. "Anger and Stress: The Role of Landscape Posters in an Office Setting." *Environment and Behavior* 40 (3): 355–81.

Lamers, F., P. van Oppen, H. C. Comijs, J. H. Smit, P. Spinhoven, A. J. van Balkom et al. 2011. "Comorbidity Patterns of Anxiety and Depressive Disorders in a Large Cohort Study: The Netherlands Study of Depression and Anxiety (NESDA)." *Journal of Clinical Psychiatry* 72 (3): 341–48.

Lazarus, A. A. 1992. "The Multimodal Approach to the Treatment of Minor Depression." *American Journal of Psychotherapy* 46 (1): 50–57.

Lazarus, R. S., and B. N. Lazarus. 1994. *Passion and Reason: Making Sense of Our Emotions.* New York: Oxford University Press.

Lebeau, R. T., C. D. Davies, N. C. Culver, and M. G. Craske. 2013. "Homework Compliance Counts in Cognitive-Behavioral Therapy." *Cognitive Behavior Therapy* 42 (3): 171–79.

LeDoux, J. 2012. "Rethinking the Emotional Brain." *Neuron* 73 (4): 653–76.

Lee, J. K., and S. M. Orsillo. 2014. "Investigating Cognitive Flexibility as a Potential Mechanism of Mindfulness in Generalized Anxiety Disorder." *Journal of Behavior Therapy and Experimental Psychiatry* 45 (1): 208–16.

Leman, M., D. Moelants, M. Varewyck, F. Styns, L. van Noorden, and J. P. Martens. 2013. "Activating and Relaxing Music Entrains the Speed of Beat Synchronized Walking." *PLoS One* 8 (7): e67932. doi: 10.1371/journal.pone.0067932.

Lench, H. C., S. A. Flores, and S. W. Bench. 2011. "Discrete Emotions Predict Changes in Cognition, Judgment, Experience, Behavior, and Physiology: A Meta-Analysis of Experimental Emotion Elicitations." *Psychological Bulletin* 137 (5): 834–55.

Leung, M. K., C. C. Chan, J. Yin, C. F. Lee, K. F. So, and T. M. Lee. 2013. "Increased Gray Matter Volume in the Right Angular and Posterior Parahippocampal Gyri in Loving-Kindness Meditators." *Social Cognitive and Affective Neuroscience* 8 (1): 34–39. doi: 10.1093/scan/nss076.

Lewis, C., J. Pearce, and J. I. Bisson. 2012. "Efficacy, Cost-Effectiveness and Acceptability of Self-Help Interventions for Anxiety Disorders: Systematic Review." *The British Journal of Psychiatry* 200 (1): 15–21.

Li, W., X. Mai, and C. Liu. 2014. "The Default Mode Network and Social Understanding of Others: What Do Brain Connectivity Studies Tell Us?" *Frontiers in Human Neuroscience* 8: 74. doi: 10.3389/fnhum.2014.00074.

Lieberman, M. D., N. I. Eisenberger, M. J. Crockett, S. M. Tom, J. H. Pfeifer, and B. M. Way. 2007. "Putting Feelings into Words: Affect Labeling Disrupts Amygdala Activity in Response to Affective Stimuli." *Psychological Science* 18 (5): 421–28.

Linares, I. M., C. Trzesniak, M. H. Chagas, J. E. Hallak, A. E. Nardi, and J. A. Crippa. 2012. "Neuroimaging in Specific Phobia Disorder: A Systematic Review of the Literature." *Revista Brasileira de Psiquiatria* 34 (1): 101–11.

Low, A. 1950. *Mental Health Through Will Training*. Boston: Christopher Publishing House.

Lua, P. L., and S. Y. Wong. 2011. "Can Dark Chocolate Alleviate Anxiety, Depressive and Stress Symptoms Among Trainee Nurses? A Parallel, Open-Label Study." *ASEAN Journal of Psychiatry* 12 (2): 157–68.

Lyubomirsky, S., L. King, and E. Diener. 2005. "The Benefits of Frequent Positive Affect: Does Happiness Lead to Success?" *Psychological Bulletin* 131 (6): 803–55.

Mahon, N. E., A. Yarcheski, T. J. Yarcheski, and M. M. Hanks. 2007. "Relations of Low Frustration Tolerance Beliefs with Stress, Depression, and Anxiety in Young Adolescents." *Psychological Reports* 100 (1): 98–100.

Mahoney, A. E., and P. M. McEvoy. 2012. "A Transdiagnostic Examination of Intolerance of Uncertainty Across Anxiety and Depressive Disorders." *Cognitive Behaviour Therapy* 41 (3): 212–22.

Malyszczak, K., T. Pawlowski, A. Pyszel, and A. Kiejna. 2006. "Correlation Between Depressive and Anxiety Symptoms, Distress, and Functioning." *Psychiatria Polska* [Psychiatric Policy] 40 (2): 269–77.

Mantar, A., B. Yemez, and T. Alkin. 2011. "Anxiety Sensitivity and Its Importance in Psychiatric Disorders." *Turkish Journal of Psychiatry* 22 (3): 187–93.

Manzoni, G. M., F. Pagnini, G. Castelnuovo, and E. Molinari. 2008. "Relaxation Training for Anxiety: A Ten-Years Systematic Review with Meta-Analysis." *BMC Psychiatry* 8: 41. doi: 10.1186/1471-244X-8-4

Mauss, I. B., A. S. Troy, and M. K. LeBourgeois. 2013. "Poorer Sleep Quality Is Associated with Lower Emotion-Regulation Ability in a Laboratory Paradigm." *Cognition and Emotion* 27 (3): 567–76.

McAndrew, F. T., S. Turner, A. C. Fiedeldey and Y. Sharma. 1998. "A Cross-Cultural Ranking of the Pleasantness of Visual and Non-Visual Features of Outdoor Environments." Paper presented at the annual meeting of the Human Behavior and Evolution Society, Davis, CA.

McEvoy, P. M., H. Watson, E. R. Watkins, and P. Nathan. 2013. "The Relationship Between Worry, Rumination, and Comorbidity: Evidence for Repetitive Negative Thinking as a Transdiagnostic Construct." *Journal of Affective Disorders* 151 (1): 313–20.

McEwen, B. S. 1998. "Protective and Damaging Effects of Stress Mediators." *New England Journal of Medicine* 338 (3): 171–79.

———. 2006. "Protective and Damaging Effects of Stress Mediators: Central Role of the Brain." *Dialogues in Clinical Neuroscience* 8 (4): 367–81.

McEwen, B. S., and J. C. Wingfield. 2003. "The Concept of Allostasis in Biology and Biomedicine." *Hormones and Behavior* 43 (1): 2–15.

McLean, C. P., A. Asnaani, B. T. Litz, and S. G. Hofmann. 2011. "Gender Differences in Anxiety Disorders: Prevalence, Course of Illness, Comorbidity and Burden of Illness." *Journal of Psychiatric Research* 45 (8): 1027–35.

McMillan, K. A., G. J. Asmundson, M. J. Zvolensky, and R. N. Carleton. 2012. "Startle Response and Anxiety Sensitivity: Subcortical Indices of Physiologic Arousal and Fear Responding." *Emotion* 12 (6): 1264–72.

Moran, J. M., W. M. Kelley, and T. F. Heatherton. 2013. "What Can the Organization of the Brain's Default Mode Network Tell Us About Self-Knowledge?" *Frontiers in Human Neuroscience* 7: 391. doi: 10.3389/fnhum.2013.00391.

Morin, A., and B. Hamper. 2012. "Self-Reflection and the Inner Voice: Activation of the Left Inferior Frontal Gyrus During Perceptual and Conceptual Self-Referential Thinking." *Open Neuroimaging Journal* 6: 78–89. doi: 10.2174/1874440001206010078.

Nechvatal, J. M., and D. M Lyons. 2013. "Coping Changes the Brain." *Frontiers in Behavioral Neuroscience* 7: 13. doi: 10.3389/fnbeh.2013.00013. Collection 2013.

Nelson, D., and C. Cooper. 2005. "Stress and Health: A Positive Direction." *Stress and Health: Journal of the International Society for the Investigation of Stress* 21 (2): 73–75.

Norton, P. J., S. A Hayes, and D. A. Hope. 2004. "Effects of a Transdiagnostic Group Treatment for Anxiety on Secondary Depression." *Depression and Anxiety* 20 (4): 198–202.

Ochsner, K. N., and J. J. Gross. 2008. "Cognitive Emotion Regulation: Insights from Social Cognitive and Affective Neuroscience." *Current Directions in Psychological Science* 17 (2): 153–58.

Olatunji, B. O., J. M. Cisler, and B. J. Deacon. 2010. "Efficacy of Cognitive Behavioral Therapy for Anxiety Disorders: A Review of Meta-Analytic Findings." *Psychiatric Clinics of North America* 33 (3): 557–77.

Olatunji, B. O., K. Naragon-Gainey, and K. B. Wolitzky-Taylor. 2013. "Specificity of Rumination in Anxiety and Depression: A Multimodal Meta-Analysis." *Clinical Psychology: Science and Practice* 20 (3): 225–57.

Olsson, A., K. I. Nearing, and E. A. Phelps. 2007. "Learning Fears by Observing Others: The Neural Systems of Social Fear Transmission." *Social Cognitive and Affective Neuroscience* 2 (1): 3–11.

Öst, L. 2008. "Cognitive Behavior Therapy for Anxiety Disorders: Forty Years of Progress." *Nordic Journal of Psychiatry* 62 (Suppl. 47): 5–10.

Otte, C. 2011. "Cognitive Behavioral Therapy in Anxiety Disorders: Current State of the Evidence." *Dialogues in Clinical Neuroscience* 13 (4): 413–21.

Pané-Farré, C. A., K. Fenske, J. P. Stender, C. Meyer, U. John, H. J. Rumpf, U. Hapke, and A. O. Hamm. 2013. "Sub-Threshold Panic Attacks and Agoraphobic Avoidance Increase Comorbidity of Mental Disorders: Results from an Adult General Population Sample." *Journal of Anxiety Disorders* 27 (5): 485–93.

Pase, M. P., A. B. Scholey, A. Pipingas, M. Kras, K. Nolidin, A. Gibbs, K. Wesnes, and C. Stough. 2013. "Cocoa Polyphenols Enhance Positive Mood States But Not Cognitive Performance: A Randomized, Placebo-Controlled Trial." *Journal of Psychopharmacology* 27 (5): 451–58.

Pavlov, I. P. 1941. *Lectures on Conditioned Reflexes.* Vol. 2 of *Conditioned Reflexes and Psychiatry,* translated and edited by W. H. Gantt. London: Lawrence and Wishart.

Pennebaker, J. W., and S. K. Beall. 1986. "Confronting a Traumatic Event: Toward an Understanding of Inhibition and Disease." *Journal of Abnormal Psychology* 95 (3): 274–81.

Penney, A. M., D. Mazmanian, and C. Rudanycz. 2013. "Comparing Positive and Negative Beliefs About Worry in Predicting Generalized Anxiety Disorder Symptoms." *Canadian Journal of Behavioural Science* 45 (1): 34–41.

Perkins, A. M., A. Cooper, M. Abdelall, L. D. Smillie, and P. J. Corr. 2010. "Personality and Defensive Reactions: Fear, Trait Anxiety, and Threat Magnification." *Journal of Personality* 78 (3): 1071–90.

Perls, F. 1973. *The Gestalt Approach and Eye Witness to Therapy.* Palo Alto: Science and Behavior Books.

Perls, F., P. Goodman, and R. Hefferline. 1951. *Gestalt Therapy: Excitement and Growth in the Human Personality.* New York: Julian Press.

Perou, R., R. H. Bitsko, S. J. Blumberg, P. Pastor, R. M. Ghandour, J. C. Gfroerer et al. 2013. "Mental Health Surveillance Among Children—United States, 2005–2011." *Morbidity and Mortality Weekly Report* 62 (Suppl. 2): 1–35.

Philippot, P., N. Vrielynck, and V. Muller. 2010. "Cognitive Processing Specificity of Anxious Apprehension: Impact on Distress and Performance During Speech Exposure." *Behavior Therapy* 41 (4): 575–86.

Piet, J., H. Würtzen, and R. Zachariae. 2012. "The Effect of Mindfulness-Based Therapy on Symptoms of Anxiety and Depression in Adult Cancer Patients and Survivors: A Systematic Review and Meta-Analysis." *Journal of Consulting and Clinical Psychology* 80 (6): 1007–20.

Popper, K. 1962. *Conjectures and Refutations: The Growth of Scientific Knowledge.* New York: Basic Books.

Posner, M. I., and M. K. Rothbart. 2007. "Research on Attention Networks as a Model for the Integration of Psychological Science." *Annual Review of Psychology* 58: 1–23.

Pothoulaki, M., R. MacDonald, and P. Flowers. 2012. "The Use of Music in Chronic Illness: Evidence and Arguments." In *Music, Health, and Wellbeing*, edited by R. A. R. MacDonald, G. Kreutz, and L. Mitchell. New York: Oxford University Press.

Querstret, D., and M. Cropley. 2013. "Assessing Treatments Used to Reduce Rumination and/or Worry: A Systematic Review." *Clinical Psychology Review* 33 (8): 996–1009.

Radhu N., Z. J. Daskalakis, C. L. Guglietti, F. Farzan, M. S. Barr, C. A. Arpin-Cribbie, P. B. Fitzgerald, and P. Ritvo. 2011. "Cognitive Behavioral Therapy-Related Increases in Cortical Inhibition in Problematic Perfectionists." *Brain Stimulation* 5 (1): 44–54.

Rayburn, N. R., and M. W. Otto. 2003. "Cognitive-Behavioral Therapy for Panic Disorder: A Review of Treatment Elements, Strategies, and Outcomes." *CNS Spectrum* 8 (5): 356–62.

Redding, R. E., E. M. Forman, B. A. Gaudiano, and J. D. Herbert. 2008. "Popular Self-Help Books for Anxiety, Depression and Trauma: How Scientifically Grounded and Useful Are They?" *Professional Psychology: Research and Practice* 39 (5): 537–45.

Reinecke, A., J. Hoyer, M. Rinck, and E. S. Becker. 2013. "Cognitive-Behavioural Therapy Reduces Unwanted Thought Intrusions in Generalized Anxiety Disorder." *Journal of Behavior Therapy and Experimental Psychiatry* 44 (1): 1–6.

Reiss, S., and R. J. McNally. 1985. "Expectancy Model of Fear." In *Theoretical Issues in Behavior Therapy*, edited by S. Reiss and R. R. Bootzin. New York: Academic Press.

Reuther, E. T., T. E. Davis, B. M. Rudy, W. S. Jenkins, S. E. Whiting, and A. C. May. 2013. "Intolerance Of Uncertainty as the Mediator of rhe Relationship Between Perfectionism and Obsessive-Compulsive Symptom Severity." *Depression and Anxiety* 30 (8): 773–77.

Richo, D. 2008. Everyday Commitments: Choosing a Life of Love, Realism, and Acceptance. Boston: Shambhala.

Riley, C., M. Lee, Z. Cooper, C. G. Fairburn, and R. Shafran. 2007. "A Randomized, Controlled Trial of Cognitive-Behaviour Therapy for Clinical Perfectionism: A Preliminary Study." *Behaviour Research and Therapy* 45 (9): 2221–31.

Rosellini, A. J., L. A. Rutter, M. L. Bourgeois, B. O. Emmert-Aronson, and T. A. Brown. 2013. "The Relevance of Age of Onset to the Psychopathology of Social Phobia." *Journal of Psychopathology and Behavioral Assessment* 35 (3): 356–65.

Sabatinelli, D., E. E. Fortune, Q. Li, A. Siddiqui, C. Krafft, W. T. Oliver, S. Beck, and J. Jeffries. 2011. "Emotional Perception: Meta-Analyses of Face and Natural Scene Processing." *Neuroimage* 54 (3): 2524–33.

Saboonchi, F., and L. G. Lundh. 2003. "Perfectionism, Anger, Somatic Health, and Positive Affect." *Personality and Individual Differences* 35 (7): 1585–99.

Salter, A. 1949. *Conditioned Reflex Therapy*. New York: Creative Age Press.

Sánchez-Meca, J., A. I. Rosa-Alcázar, F. Marín-Martínez, and A. Gómez-Conesa. 2010. "Psychological Treatment of Panic Disorder with or Without Agoraphobia: A Meta-Analysis." *Clinical Psychology Review* 30 (1): 37–50.

Sassaroli, S., L. J. R. Lauro, G. M. Ruggiero, M. C. Mauri, P. Vinai, and R. Frost. 2008. "Perfectionism in Depression, Obsessive-Compulsive Disorder and Eating Disorders." *Behaviour Research and Therapy* 46 (6): 757–65.

Schachter, S., and J. Singer. 1962. "Cognitive, Social, and Physiological Determinants of Emotional State." *Psychological Review* 69 (5): 397–99.

Schweckendiek J., T. Klucken, C. J. Merz, K. Tabbert, B. Walter, W. Ambach, D. Vaitl, and R. Stark. 2011. "Weaving the (Neuronal) Web: Fear Learning in Spider Phobia." *Neuroimage* 54 (1): 681–88.

Scott, K. M., M. Von Korff, J. Alonso, M. Angermeyer, E. J. Bromet, R. Bruffaerts et al. 2008. "Age Patterns in the Prevalence of DSM-IV Depressive/Anxiety Disorders with and Without Physical Co-Morbidity." *Psychological Medicine* 38 (11): 1659–69.

Seery M. D., M. Weisbuch, M. A. Hetenyi, and J. Blascovich. 2010. "Cardiovascular Measures Independently Predict Performance in a University Course." *Psychophysiology* 47 (3): 535–39.

Seih, Y. T., C. K. Chung, and J. W. Pennebaker. 2011. "Experimental Manipulations of Perspective Taking and Perspective Switching in Expressive Writing." *Cognition and Emotion* 25 (5): 926–38.

Siev, J., and D. L. Chambless. 2007. "Specificity of Treatment Effects: Cognitive Therapy and Relaxation for Generalized Anxiety and Panic Disorders." *Journal of Consulting and Clinical Psychology* 75 (4): 513–22.

Spielberg, J. M., A. A. De Leon, K. Bredemeier, W. Heller, A. S. Engels, S. L. Warren, L. D. Crocker, B. P. Sutton, and G. A Miller. 2013. "Anxiety Type Modulates Immediate Versus Delayed Engagement of Attention-Related Brain Regions." *Brain and Behavior* 3 (5): 532–551.

Stamps, A. E. 3rd. 1990. "Use of Photographs to Simulate Environments: A Meta-Analysis." *Perceptual and Motor Skills* 71 (3): 907–13.

———. 2008. "Some Findings on Prospect and Refuge Theory: II." *Perceptual and Motor Skills* 107 (1): 141–58.

———. 2010. "Use of Static and Dynamic Media to Simulate Environments: A Meta-Analysis." *Perceptual and Motor Skills* 111 (2): 355–64.

———. 2012. "How Distance Mitigates Perceived Threat at 30–90 M." *Perceptual and Motor Skills* 114 (3): 709–16.

Stockdale, B. 2011. "Writing in Physical and Concomitant Mental Illness: Biological Underpinnings and Applications for Practice." In *Research on Writing Approaches in Mental Health. Studies in Writing*, edited by L. L'Abate and L. G. Sweeney. Bingley, United Kingdom: Emerald Group Publishing.

Thoma, M. V., R. La Marca, R. Brönnimann, L. Finkel, U. Ehlert, and U. M. Nater. 2013. "The Effect of Music on the Human Stress Response." *PLoS One* 8 (8): e70156. doi: 10.1371/journal.pone.0070156.

Trappe, H. J. 2009. "Music and Health—What Kind of Music Is Helpful for Whom? What Music not?" *Deutsche Medizinische Wochenschrift* 134 (51–52): 2601–6 (Article in German).

Ulrich, R. S 1977. "Visual Landscape Preference: A Model and Application." *Man-Environment Systems* 7 (5): 279–93.

van der Zwaag, M. D., C. Dijksterhuis, D. de Waard, B. L. Mulder, J. H. Westerink, and K. A. Brookhuis. 2012. "The Influence of Music on Mood and Performance While Driving." *Ergonomics* 55 (1): 12–22.

van der Zwaag, M. D., J. H. Janssen, C. Nass, J. H. Westerink, S. Chowdhury, and D. de Waard. 2013. "Using Music to Change Mood While Driving." *Ergonomics* 56 (10): 1504–14.

van Emmerik, A. A., J. H. Kamphuis, and P. M. Emmelkamp. 2008. "Treating Acute Stress Disorder and Posttraumatic Stress Disorder with Cognitive Behavioral Therapy or Structured Writing Therapy: A Randomized Controlled Trial." *Psychotherapy and Psychosomatics* 77 (2): 93–100.

Velarde, M. D., G. Fry, and M. Tveit 2007. "Health Effects of Viewing Landscapes—Landscape Types in Environmental Psychology." *Urban Forestry and Urban Greening* 6 (4): 199–212.

Völler, H. 2006. "Significance of Changes in Habits Followed by Risk Reduction." *Clinical Research in Cardiology* 95 (Suppl. 6): V16–11.

Von Clausewitz, C. 1982. *On War.* New York: Penguin.

Walther, D. B., E. Caddigan, L. Fei-Fei, and D. M. Beck. 2009. "Natural Scene Categories Revealed in Distributed Patterns of Activity in the Human Brain." *Journal of Neuroscience* 29 (34): 10573–81.

Watson, D., and Kendall, P. C. 1989. "Understanding Anxiety and Depression: Their Relation to Negative and Positive Affective States." In *Anxiety and Depression: Distinctive and Overlapping Features*, edited by P. C. Kendall and D. Watson. San Diego, CA: Academic Press.

Weich, S., H. L. Pearce, P. Croft, S. Singh, I. Crome, J. Bashford, and M. Frisher. 2014. "Effect of Anxiolytic and Hypnotic Drug Prescriptions on Mortality Hazards: Retrospective Cohort Study." *British Medical Journal* 348: g1996. http://www.bmj.com/content/348/bmj.g1996.

Williams, T. 1974. *The Glass Menagerie.* New York: New Directions.

Wolitzky-Taylor, K. B., N. Castriotta, E. J. Lenze, M. A. Stanley, and M. G. Craske. 2010. "Anxiety Disorders in Older Adults: A Comprehensive Review." *Depression and Anxiety* 27 (2): 190–211.

Wolpe, Joseph. 1967. Lecture given at Temple University, Philadelphia, PA.

Xu, Y., F. Schneier, R. G. Heimberg, K. Princisvalle, M. R. Liebowitz, S. Wang, and C. Blanco. 2012. "Gender Differences in Social Anxiety Disorder: Results from the National Epidemiologic Sample on Alcohol and Related Conditions." *Journal of Anxiety Disorders* 26 (1): 12–19.

Yang, C. M., and F. C. Hsiao. 2012. "Management of Sleep Disorders—Cognitive Behavioral Therapy for Insomnia." In *Introduction to Modern Sleep Technology*, edited by R. P. Chiang and S. Kang. New York: Springer Science + Business Media.

William J. Knaus, EdD, is a licensed psychologist with more than forty years of clinical experience in working with people suffering from anxiety and depression. He has appeared on numerous regional and national television shows including *Today*, and more than one hundred radio shows. His ideas have appeared in national magazines such as *U.S. News and World Report* and *Good Housekeeping*, and major newspapers such as the *Washington Post* and the *Chicago Tribune*. He is one of the original directors of training in rational emotive behavior therapy (REBT). Knaus is author of twenty books, including *The Cognitive Behavioral Workbook for Anxiety*, *The Cognitive Behavioral Workbook for Depression*, and *The Procrastination Workbook*.

Foreword writer **Jon Carlson, PsyD, EdD, ABPP**, is distinguished professor in the division of psychology and counseling at Governors State University, IL.

Index

FROM OUR PUBLISHER—

As the publisher at New Harbinger and a clinical psychologist since 1978, I know that emotional problems are best helped with evidence-based therapies. These are the treatments derived from scientific research (randomized controlled trials) that show what works. Whether these treatments are delivered by trained clinicians or found in a self-help book, they are designed to provide you with proven strategies to overcome your problem.

Therapies that aren't evidence-based—whether offered by clinicians or in books—are much less likely to help. In fact, therapies that aren't guided by science may not help you at all. That's why this New Harbinger book is based on scientific evidence that the treatment can relieve emotional pain.

This is important: if this book isn't enough, and you need the help of a skilled therapist, use the following resources to find a clinician trained in the evidence-based protocols appropriate for your problem. And if you need more support—a community that understands what you're going through and can show you ways to cope—resources for that are provided below, as well.

Real help is available for the problems you have been struggling with. The skills you can learn from evidence-based therapies will change your life.

Matthew McKay, PhD
Publisher, New Harbinger Publications

**If you need a therapist, the following organization
can help you find a therapist trained in cognitive behavioral therapy (CBT).**

The Association for Behavioral & Cognitive Therapies (ABCT) Find-a-Therapist service offers a list of therapists schooled in CBT techniques. Therapists listed are licensed professionals who have met the membership requirements of ABCT and who have chosen to appear in the directory.

Please visit www.abct.org and click on *Find a Therapist*.

**For additional support for patients, family, and friends,
please contact the following:**

Anxiety and Depression Association of American (ADAA)
please visit www.adaa.org

National Alliance on Mental Illness (NAMI)
please visit www.nami.org

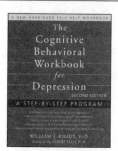
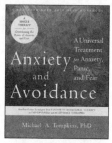
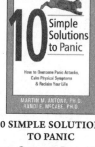
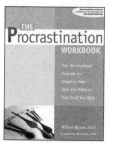
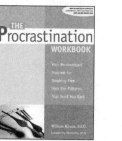
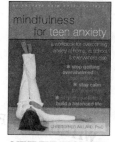

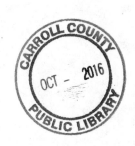